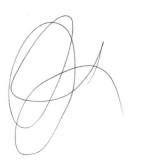

Treatment of Late-Life Depression, Anxiety, Trauma, and Substance Abuse

Treatment of Late-Life Depression, Anxiety, Trauma, and Substance Abuse

EDITED BY PATRICIA A. AREÁN

American Psychological Association • Washington, DC

Published by
American Psychological Association
750 First Street, NE
Washington, DC 20002
www.apa.org

To order
APA Order Department
P.O. Box 92984
Washington, DC 20090-2984
Tel: (800) 374-2721; Direct: (202) 336-5510
Fax: (202) 336-5502; TDD/TTY: (202) 336-6123
Online: www.apa.org/pubs/books
E-mail: order@apa.org

In the U.K., Europe, Africa, and the Middle East, copies may be ordered from
American Psychological Association
3 Henrietta Street
Covent Garden, London
WC2E 8LU England

Typeset in Goudy by Circle Graphics, Inc., Columbia, MD

Printer: Maple Press, York, PA
Cover Designer: Mercury Publishing Services, Inc., Rockville, MD

The opinions and statements published are the responsibility of the authors, and such opinions and statements do not necessarily represent the policies of the American Psychological Association. Any views expressed in chapter 5 do not necessarily represent the views of the United States government, and the author's participation in the work is not meant to serve as an official endorsement.

Library of Congress Cataloging-in-Publication Data

Treatment of late-life depression, anxiety, trauma, and substance abuse / edited by Patricia A. Areán. — First edition.
    pages cm
  Includes bibliographical references and index.
  ISBN-13: 978-1-4338-1839-4
  ISBN-10: 1-4338-1839-6
  1. Psychotherapy for older people. 2. Older people—Psychology. 3. Older people—Mental health. 4. Geriatric psychiatry. I. Areán, Patricia A.
  RC480.54.T74 2015
  616.89'140846—dc23
                              2014019617

British Library Cataloguing-in-Publication Data
A CIP record is available from the British Library.

Printed in the United States of America
First Edition

http://dx.doi.org/10.1037/14524-000

CONTENTS

CONTRIBUTORS

Patricia A. Areán, PhD, Department of Psychiatry, University of California, San Francisco

Catherine Ayers, PhD, ABPP, VA San Diego Healthcare System and Department of Psychiatry, University of California, San Diego

Joan M. Cook, PhD, Department of Psychiatry, Yale School of Medicine, New Haven, CT, and Evaluation Division, National Center for PTSD, West Haven, CT

Rebecca M. Crabb, PhD, National Network of PST Clinicians, Trainers, and Researchers, San Francisco, CA

Elizabeth A. DiNapoli, MA, Department of Psychology, University of Alabama, Tuscaloosa

Stephanie Dinnen, MS, Department of Psychiatry, Yale School of Medicine, New Haven, CT

Michael LaRocca, MA, Department of Psychology, University of Alabama, Tuscaloosa

Amy Leibowitz, PsyD, Division of Research, Kaiser Permanente Northern California, and private psychotherapy practice, Oakland, CA

Nancy H. Liu, PhD, Department of Medicine, University of California, San Francisco

Nicole S. MacFarland, PhD, Executive Director, Senior Hope Counseling Inc., Albany, NY

Sara Honn Qualls, PhD, Psychology Department, University of Colorado, Colorado Springs

Patrick J. Raue, PhD, Department of Psychiatry, Weill Cornell Medical College, New York, NY

Derek D. Satre, PhD, Department of Psychiatry, University of California, San Francisco, and Division of Research, Kaiser Permanente Northern California, Oakland

Jason M. Satterfield, PhD, Department of Medicine, University of California, San Francisco

Lawrence Schonfeld, PhD, Louis de la Parte Florida Mental Health Institute, University of South Florida, Tampa

Forrest Scogin, PhD, Department of Psychology, University of Alabama, Tuscaloosa

Katrina Strickland, MA, VA San Diego Healthcare System, San Diego, CA

Julie Loebach Wetherell, PhD, VA San Diego Healthcare System and Department of Psychiatry, University of California, San Diego

Treatment of Late-Life Depression, Anxiety, Trauma, and Substance Abuse

INTRODUCTION

PATRICIA A. AREÁN

I am often asked how I became interested in working with older adults. Back in the early 1980s, I was employed as a behavioral technologist at Goldwater Memorial Hospital in New York City, a public sector rehabilitation and skilled nursing facility. I actually had two jobs, one as a research assistant working on a project to study biofeedback and occupational therapy with people who had had a stroke, and one as a "friendly visitor"—an assistant to a clinical psychologist treating depression in nursing home residents by using group therapy models. Most of the patients at Goldwater were over the age of 60, and many had disabilities that kept them from being able to live on their own. Although the administration at Goldwater did all they could to make the hospital cheery, it was still a skilled nursing facility, and the constant reminders about limited function and the need for 24/7 care were hard to ignore.

http://dx.doi.org/10.1037/14524-001
Treatment of Late-Life Depression, Anxiety, Trauma, and Substance Abuse, P. A. Areán (Editor)

My first friendly visitor patient (whom I will call Daisy) was an older woman with Guillain-Barré syndrome, a progressive polyneuropathy that results in a progressive paralysis that eventually remits; people who have Guillain-Barré often recover and regain full use of their functions. Daisy, however, still had a partial disability, having only regained partial use of her arms, and was completely paralyzed from the hips down. She had been referred to one of the psychotherapy groups after the recent onset of depression following an incident in which the nursing staff had accidently dropped Daisy in the shower and could not help her back up into her wheelchair (Daisy weighed about 300 pounds). Daisy had not been responding well to the group and refused to participate in the discussions. I was asked to meet with her one-on-one to help figure out how we could best help her with her depression. At the time, Drs. Dolores and Larry Thompson had begun to publish data from their research on cognitive behavior therapy (CBT; see Chapter 2, this volume) in late-life depression, with very promising results indicating that CBT was an effective behavioral intervention. With permission from my supervisor, I decided to try CBT with Daisy, starting with behavioral activation and eventually moving to cognitive reappraisal. Within a matter of 3 weeks, Daisy had changed radically. Having been initially uncommunicative and apathetic, she began to become more involved in activities around the hospital, and she joined a patient advocates group. By 6 weeks, she was laughing with me and sharing anecdotes of her life, while also sharing how hard it was for her to have been healthy her whole life and suddenly become so dependent on other people. By the end of 6 months, Daisy no longer needed to stay at Goldwater, having advocated for a move to a more comfortable residential care facility. Before my eyes, I saw a gray, dejected women turn into a sunny, beautiful, and independent person. I could see in her eyes what she must have been like when she was younger and that that person was still there, deep down, and could live a happy life despite her circumstances. In essence, I owe my career in geropsychology to Daisy, and to the patients I worked with subsequently.

WHAT EXACTLY DOES "OLDER ADULT" MEAN?

Age 65 is generally agreed to be the age at which a person is considered "old." Historically, older age has been associated with declining physical and cognitive health, fragility, and proximity to the end of life. At the time that this age definition was set—in the late 1800s—few people lived past the age of 65, and those around that age were very frail (Global Age-Watch Administration, 2013). However, today, although people over 65 are still referred to as "older adults," people can expect to live far past this age; in fact, the average age of mortality overall in the United States is 79 (Gallo et al.,

2013). Research shows that people in their 60s and 70s are, on average quite healthy; although the risks for chronic illnesses and cognitive impairments do increase with age, working with older adults is no longer equivalent to working with people who are frail or have a disability (Lacey, Belcher, & Croft, 2013). In fact, professionals working with older adults can expect to encounter a heterogeneous population whose members have a vast fund of experience and knowledge that makes working with them a unique experience.

AN AGING AMERICA

According to the Centers for Disease Control and Prevention and the World Health Organization, this is the first time in history that people over the age of 65 outnumber people under the age of 5 (Kowal et al., 2012). This increase is due in part to improved health care at younger ages, better nutrition, and better acute and chronic illness management (Clarke et al., 2012).

Although older adults are healthier, they still require specialized health and mental health care. However, the geriatric medicine and geropsychology workforce has not kept up with the growth in older populations; as a result, there will likely be a significant crisis in the health care world (Bartels & Naslund, 2013). For psychology, this means that clinicians will see a growing number of older patients in their practice but will have very little experience in the best methods for working with this unique population. Although mental disorders are not as common in later life as they are in younger populations (assuming a survival aspect to aging in general; Mezuk & Kendler, 2012), they can be very disabling and costly. It is a little-known fact that older adults with depression, anxiety, and alcohol misuse are more likely to complete suicide than any other age group (Caine & Conwell, 2001; Shah, 2010), have more disabilities (as a group), and have higher medical costs than older adults without mental disorders (Katon, Lin, Russo, & Unützer, 2003; Unützer, Bruce, & Workgroup, 2002; see also the Institute of Medicine's, 2012, recommendations on the mental health and substance abuse workforce for older adults).

OLDER ADULTS DO RESPOND TO PSYCHOTHERAPY

When I was a student in the 1980s, there was a common belief in community mental health that older adults could not benefit from psychotherapy and that, in general, older adults would prefer a medication to talk therapy. Over the past 25 years, these assumptions have been widely dispelled. As for treatment preference, older adults are more likely to prefer talk therapies and less likely to ask for medication (Raue, Schulberg, Heo, Klimstra, & Bruce,

2009). This preference may be in some way a result of the relative effect of treatment options. According to a number of meta-analyses, antidepressant medication for late-life depression is less effective than psychotherapy, and according to a recent meta-analysis (Nelson & Devanand, 2011), only one in 10 older adults will experience an improvement from antidepressants. However, a recent large clinical trial demonstrated that one in four older adults respond to psychotherapy (Areán et al., 2010). Not only is psychotherapy the more effective treatment option for older adults but its effects are as good as those seen in younger adults. According to Cuijpers, van Straten, Smit, and Andersson (2009), psychotherapy results in moderate effects in treatment in both younger and older adults.

WHY DO CLINICAL PSYCHOLOGISTS NEED THIS BOOK?

Clearly, anyone providing psychotherapy will need to be prepared for the multitude of older adults seeking help. This book is meant to be a compendium of information on best practices in treating mental disorders in late life. The primary audience for this book consists of psychologists, social workers, and psychiatrists who use psychosocial interventions as part of their practice. Other readers who might benefit from the material herein include other professionals who interact with older adults in their practice, such as physical therapists. This book addresses many of the questions the chapter authors and I are asked by professionals and students interested in working with older adults: What do I need to know about older adults to work effectively with them? What issues do we need to consider when making a diagnosis? What are the evidence-based treatments for geriatric mental disorders, and how are they adapted for older age?

To address these questions, we begin with an overview of geropsychology and the competencies psychologists need to work with older adults. In Chapter 1, Sara Honn Qualls covers the competencies needed to work with a geriatric population. The next three chapters focus on evidence-based practices for treating depression. The interventions were selected on the basis of common agreement among meta-analytic and systematic reviews that the evidence base is sufficient to recommend them as frontline psychotherapies. Elizabeth A. DiNapoli, Michael LaRocca, and Forrest Scogin focus on cognitive behavior treatment approaches in Chapter 2. In Chapter 3, Patrick J. Raue and I focus on interpersonal psychotherapy for older adults, and in Chapter 4, Rebecca M. Crabb and I cover the use of problem-solving therapy. Chapter 5, by Catherine Ayers, Katrina Strickland, and Julie Loebach Wetherell, and Chapter 6, by Joan M. Cook and Stephanie Dinnen, describe treatments for anxiety and trauma disorders. These chapters review the most common interventions for these disorders and provide recommendations as to the best treatments. Finally, Chapters 7 through 9 focus on psycho-social interventions for substance abuse disorders. Derek D. Satre and Amy Leibowitz (Chapter 7) discuss the use of relapse prevention therapy for substance use in older adults. In Chapter 8, Nancy H. Liu and Jason M. Satterfield focus on the use of the screening, brief intervention, and referral-to-treatment model, which is a stepped-care model of substance use commonly used in primary care settings. In Chapter 9, Lawrence Schonfeld and Nicole S. MacFarland focus on the use of motivational interviewing and its application to older adults.

The section titled "Additional Resources for Clinicians" provides training resources to help clinicians improve their skills in working with older adults. The resources include books they might recommend to clients to complement treatment, videos illustrating how to deliver therapy, and information on continuing education and certifications in the field of geriatric psychology.

Although most chapters discuss theory to some degree, the focus of this book is practical, and the intent is to give the reader enough information to know how to work effectively with older adults. Each author provides an overview of the disorder the chapter addresses and offers a detailed case example to give the reader a how-to experience. The chapter authors and I hope that this book inspires clinicians to expand their skill set in working with older adults. We have found it rewarding to work with this wonderful population, and we seek to highlight the breadth of life experience and the depth of knowledge older adults bring to the psychotherapy endeavor.

CURRENT STATUS OF TREATMENT, ACCESS TO CARE, AND TRAINING

As is noted throughout this book, although there have been a number of accommodations to account for cognitive impairment and disability, more research is needed to determine whether these accommodations are sufficient in addressing the needs of older adults with disabilities. We have also made sure that the information provided in each chapter is based on current changes to the *Diagnostic and Statistical Manual of Mental Disorders* (5th ed.; American Psychiatric Association, 2013), and anticipated changes in the next edition of the *International Classification of Diseases* (see World Health Organization, n.d.). In addition, as researchers' understanding of the root causes of mental disorders improves, through initiatives such as the National Institute of Mental Health Research Domain Criteria Project (Cuthbert & Insel, 2013; Insel et al., 2010), they may find that intervention effectiveness is not bound to disorders but rather addresses the commonalities that are shared between disorders. As Ayers and coauthors point out in Chapter 5, problem-solving therapy, an evidence-based treatment for late-life depression, may be especially effective for older adults with generalized anxiety disorder, particularly those who show executive impairments.

Of particular interest recently is the use of technology to enhance treatment effectiveness. As an example, older adults who have access to a cell phone may benefit from text messaging reminders from therapists to complete action plans or to simply rate their mood in real time. Online versions of cognitive behavior therapy, behavioral activation therapy, and problem-solving therapy exist and may facilitate access to these effective treatments for older adults. Although older adults are less likely to own smartphones (Hafeez-Baig & Gururajan, 2010), they are a large market for smart tablets (e.g., iPads), laptop computers, and mobile devices (e.g., FitBit; PewInternet, 2013). They are also consumers of cognitive training games (e.g., Lumosity; Keenan, 2009), and preliminary evidence suggests that these games can effectively improve older adults' cognition (Anguera et al., 2013). To be seen, however, is whether these games can enhance the psychotherapy experience.

Even if interventions work, older adults still face the problem of access to quality care. Because few training programs offer training in geropsychology, clinicians now—and in the future—will be unprepared to meet the needs of older clients. As Qualls points out in Chapter 1, they will need to learn several competencies to be effective with their older clients. Older adults are not simply adults who are older, and clinicians will need to know the medical, cognitive, and societal nuances of working with an older population. Fortunately, many good resources are available to help clinicians learn how to do psychotherapy with older populations; some of these resources are provided in the Additional Resources for Clinicians. In addition, the American Psychological Association is developing a consultation model for clinicians who find themselves working more and more with older adults and want advice and guidance from geropsychologists. Large medical centers, such as the one at the University of California, San Francisco, are also working to develop distance learning modules and telemedicine methods for providing expert guidance to clinicians working with older adults. With this book, we hope to inspire clinicians to learn more about working with older clients.

REFERENCES

American Psychiatric Association. (2013). *Diagnostic and statistical manual of mental disorders* (5th ed.). Washington, DC: Author.

Anguera, J. A., Boccanfuso, J., Rintoul, J. L., Al-Hashimi, O., Faraji, F., Janowich, J., . . . Gazzaley, A. (2013, September 5). Video game training enhances cognitive control in older adults. *Nature, 501,* 97–101. doi:10.1038/nature12486

Areán, P. A., Raue, P., Mackin, R. S., Kanellopoulos, D., McCulloch, C., & Alexopoulos, G. S. (2010). Problem-solving therapy and supportive therapy in older adults with major depression and executive dysfunction. *The American Journal of Psychiatry, 167*, 1391–1398. doi:10.1176/appi.ajp.2010.09091327

Bartels, S. J., & Naslund, J. A. (2013). The underside of the silver tsunami—Older adults and mental health care. *The New England Journal of Medicine, 368*, 493–496. doi:10.1056/NEJMp1211456

Caine, E. D., & Conwell, Y. (2001). Suicide in the elderly. *International Clinical Psychopharmacology, 16*(Suppl. 2), 25–30. doi:10.1097/00004850-200103002-00005

Clarke, P. M., Walter, S. J., Hayen, A., Mallon, W. J., Heijmans, J., & Studdert, D. M. (2012). Survival of the fittest: Retrospective cohort study of the longevity of Olympic medallists in the modern era. *British Medical Journal, 345*, e8308. doi:10.1136/bmj.e8308

Cuijpers, P., van Straten, A., Smit, F., & Andersson, G. (2009). Is psychotherapy for depression equally effective in younger and older adults? A meta-regression analysis. *International Psychogeriatrics, 21*, 16–24. doi:10.1017/S1041610208008089

Cuthbert, B. N., & Insel, T. R. (2013). Toward the future of psychiatric diagnosis: The seven pillars of RDoC. *BMC Medicine, 11*, 126. doi:10.1186/1741-7015-11-126

Gallo, J. J., Morales, K. H., Bogner, H. R., Raue, P. J., Zee, J., Bruce, M. L., & Reynolds, C. F., III. (2013). Long-term effect of depression care management on mortality in older adults: Follow-up of cluster randomized clinical trial in primary care. *British Medical Journal, 346.* doi:10.1136/bmj.f2570

Global Age-Watch Administration, S. S. (2013). *Frequently asked questions.* Retrieved from http://www.ssa.gov/history/age65.html

Hafeez-Baig, A., & Gururajan, R. (2010). Key common determinants for adoption of wireless technology in healthcare for India and Pakistan: Development of a conceptual model. *Studies in Health Technology and Informatics, 160*(Pt 1), 342–346.

Insel, T., Cuthbert, B., Garvey, M., Heinssen, R., Pine, D. S., Quinn, K., . . . Wang, P. (2010). Research domain criteria (RDoC): Toward a new classification framework for research on mental disorders. *The American Journal of Psychiatry, 167*, 748–751. doi:10.1176/appi.ajp.2010.09091379

Institute of Medicine. (2012). *The mental health and substance use workforce for older adults: In whose hands?* Retrieved from http://www.iom.edu/~/media/Files/Report%20Files/2012/The-Mental-Health-and-Substance-Use-Workforce-for-Older-Adults/MHSU_insert.pdf

Katon, W. J., Lin, E., Russo, J., & Unützer, J. (2003). Increased medical costs of a population-based sample of depressed elderly patients. *Archives of General Psychiatry, 60*, 897–903. doi:10.1001/archpsyc.60.9.897

Keenan, T. (2009). *Internet use in the elderly.* Retrieved from http://assets.aarp.org/rgcenter/general/bulletin_internet_09.pdf

Kowal, P., Chatterji, S., Naidoo, N., Biritwum, R., Fan, W., Lopez Ridaura, R., . . . Collaborators, S. (2012). Data resource profile: The World Health Organization

Study on global AGEing and adult health (SAGE). *International Journal of Epidemiology, 41,* 1639–1649. doi:10.1093/ije/dys210

Lacey, R. J., Belcher, J., & Croft, P. R. (2013). Does life course socioeconomic position influence chronic disabling pain in older adults? A general population study. *European Journal of Public Health, 23,* 534–540. doi:10.1093/eurpub/cks056

Mezuk, B., & Kendler, K. S. (2012). Examining variation in depressive symptoms over the life course: A latent class analysis. *Psychological Medicine, 42,* 2037–2046. doi:10.1017/S003329171200027X

Nelson, J. C., & Devanand, D. P. (2011). A systematic review and meta-analysis of placebo-controlled antidepressant studies in people with depression and dementia. *Journal of the American Geriatrics Society, 59,* 577–585. doi:10.1111/j.1532-5415.2011.03355.x

PewInternet. (2013). *Older adults and internet use.* Retrieved from http://www.pewinternet.org/Reports/2012/Older-adults-and-internet-use.aspx

Raue, P. J., Schulberg, H. C., Heo, M., Klimstra, S., & Bruce, M. L. (2009). Patients' depression treatment preferences and initiation, adherence, and outcome: A randomized primary care study. *Psychiatric Services, 60,* 337–343. doi:10.1176/appi.ps.60.3.337

Shah, A. (2010). Old age psychiatry and geriatric medicine admissions and elderly suicide rates in England. *International Psychogeriatrics, 22,* 502–504. doi:10.1017/S1041610209991700

Unützer, J., Bruce, M. L., & Workgroup, N. A. D. (2002). The elderly. *Mental Health Services Research, 4,* 245–247. doi:10.1023/A:1020924901595

World Health Organization. (n.d.). *Classifications.* Retrieved from http://www.who.int/classifications/icd/en/

1

BUILDING COMPETENCIES IN PROFESSIONAL GEROPSYCHOLOGY: GUIDELINES, TRAINING MODEL, AND STRATEGIES FOR PROFESSIONAL DEVELOPMENT

SARA HONN QUALLS

The evidence-based practice models and strategies outlined in this book are among the many competencies needed by psychologists who work with older adults. In this chapter, I describe the Pikes Peak model [PPM] for training in professional geropsychology (Knight, Karel, Hinrichsen, Qualls, & Duffy, 2009). The model comprises the categories of attitudes, knowledge, and skills, within which are 65 competencies that offer detailed guidance for psychologists who work with older adults.

WHAT DO PSYCHOLOGISTS NEED TO KNOW TO WORK WITH OLDER ADULTS?

Momentum to define what is distinct about working with older adults has built over the 30-year period since the initial training conferences referred to as Older Boulder I and II (Knight, Teri, Wohlford, & Santos,

http://dx.doi.org/10.1037/14524-002
Treatment of Late-Life Depression, Anxiety, Trauma, and Substance Abuse, P. A. Areán (Editor)

1995; Santos & VandenBos, 1982), which culminated in the conference that generated the PPM. Along the way, the literature on geropsychology, including professional geropsychology, has grown substantially, and a wealth of resource materials is now available for professionals wishing to expand, update, or specialize their practice. The Office on Aging within the American Psychological Association (APA) coordinates resources and, in coordination with APA's (n.d.) Division 20, has stimulated development of multiple resources. In addition, APA's (2014) recently revised *Guidelines for Psychological Practice With Older Adults* details distinct aspects of practice within six categories: (a) competence in and attitudes toward working with older adults; (b) general knowledge about adult development, aging, and older adults; (c) clinical issues; (d) assessment; (e) intervention, consultation, and other services; and (f) professional issues and education. Professionals seeking to build competence in working with older adults need to study these guidelines in detail as background for the specific competencies outlined in the PPM and discussed here.

Two common themes are woven through the plethora of materials and models in geropsychology. First, the biopsychosocial model of health and wellness (Engel, 1977; Frankel, Quill, & McDaniel, 2003) is embraced almost universally. Older adults' mental health is viewed in the context of the whole person, including biological aspects of health and functioning; psychological aspects, such as cognition, coping, psychopathology, and personality; and social contexts of aging (Segal, Qualls, & Smyer, 2011). Geropsychologists recognize and address the complexities caused by comorbidities and life-span contexts, among other factors. The long life of a person before he or she sees a geropsychologist is filled with normative and nonnormative events, historical and cohort influences, choices, and patterns that are critical components of any conceptualization of the person's current circumstances and needs (Baltes, Lindenberger, & Staudinger, 1998). Implementation of evidence-based protocols for treatment of psychopathology benefits from case conceptualization from a biopsychosocial model.

The second major theme, indicated in the first, is that intervention success is all about *context*. Contextual factors are as varied as the therapist–patient/client relationship (Knight, 2004) and the political and fiscal context of Medicare that defines which intervention services can be reimbursed (Karlin & Humphries, 2007). Geropsychologists work in integrated care settings across the continuum of health and wellness services from senior centers to long-term care. The context is sufficiently powerful that therapists often find it necessary to adapt the protocol that was tested in a clinical trial to meet the needs of the person in the particular context (Scogin & Shah, 2012).

THE PIKES PEAK MODEL FOR TRAINING
IN PROFESSIONAL GEROPSYCHOLOGY

A training model to guide practitioners and professional trainers extends beyond a general description of content by outlining the specific attitudes, knowledge, and skill competencies that are needed, along with the processes by which they can be acquired (Kaslow, 2004; Rodolfa et al., 2005). *Competencies* are professional behaviors that are measurable and relate to outcomes in patient well-being. Many specialty fields within psychology have adopted the competencies approach to creating a training model, including child clinical psychology (Jackson, Wu, Aylward, & Roberts, 2012), clinical health psychology (France et al., 2008), clinical neuropsychology (Hannay et al., 1998; Rey-Casserly, Roper, & Bauer, 2012), and forensic psychology (Varela & Conroy, 2012), among others. The competency approach builds off Rodolfa et al.'s (2005) cube model, which illustrates the three axes of foundational competencies, functional competencies, and steps in the training career. Training models guide the development and delivery of curricula in scope and sequential presentation, evaluation standards and strategies, and goals and strategies for supervised practice for all levels of training, from predoctoral to postlicensure.

The PPM applies the principles and processes used by other specialties to its own training models. The resulting competencies approach is relevant to practitioners as well as to students in the preprofessional pipeline. Rather than prescribing a single pathway to specialization that begins in graduate school, the PPM acknowledges that practitioners take many pathways into geropsychology, only some of which begin during formal training. Although some students commit to specialization in geropsychology early in their training career, many professionals recognize the need for more training and career preparation to work with older adults long after formal training has ended. Thus, the PPM invites established professionals to self-assess their competencies, using a tool that can be also used by supervisors or trainers (Karel, Emery, & Molinari, 2010; Karel et al., 2012).

COMPETENCIES FOR PRACTICE IN
PROFESSIONAL GEROPSYCHOLOGY

The PPM specifies four attitude competencies, 20 knowledge competencies, and 41 skill competencies, as detailed in Appendix 1.1. The *attitude* competencies include examples such as the recognition of how one's own attitudes and beliefs about aging are relevant to professional services, and the engagement in increasing one's knowledge and skills with regard to practice with older adults.

The *knowledge* competencies are divided into four groups. Group A relates to general knowledge about adult development, aging, and the older adult. Included here are knowledge about theories and research methodologies for studying typical aging, demographics, facts about biopsychosocial aging processes and norms, and awareness of diversity within the aging population. Group B focuses on foundations of clinical practice with older adults, including topics such as neuroscience, functional aging, the salience of person–environment interaction, psychopathology, and the importance and impact of health conditions. Group C addresses foundations of assessment of older adults, including theory and research on assessment of older adults, limitations in the use of assessment tools developed for younger populations with older adults, and knowledge of contextual issues relevant to assessment of older adults. Group D addresses foundations of intervention, consultation, and other services. Examples of competencies addressed in Group D are theory and practice of intervention methods for older adults specifically, issues related to delivery of services in particular settings and with other disciplines, ethics, and knowledge of health and other community services relevant to older adult clients or patients and their families.

Skill competencies are the largest group in the PPM, with 41 competencies organized within five groups. Group A contains competencies related to professional geropsychology functioning, considered foundational competencies. Examples from this group include skills in applying ethical and legal standards to aging-related clinical issues (e.g., informed consent, capacity, elder abuse); cultural and individual diversity; biopsychosocial issues; and documentation, billing, and reimbursement procedures (e.g., Medicare, Medicaid). Examples of competencies in Group B that focus on assessment include skills that address challenging differential diagnostic issues that are common in older adults, appropriate use of screening instruments, evaluation of decision-making and functional capacities or risk, and effective communication of results to stakeholders. Group C competencies are intervention skills; examples include applying appropriate modifications to existing evidence-based approaches to address biopsychosocial functioning of older adults, demonstrating the ability to implement interventions in settings where older adults receive services, and using late-life interventions. Group D competencies relate to consultation and training, and examples include consulting with staff, professionals, programs, and families; offering training related to geropsychology to other disciplines; and collaborating and coordinating across agencies and organizations. Group E contains skill competencies related to delivery of services in different settings, including outpatient and inpatient mental health settings, primary care, inpatient medical services, hospice, forensic settings, and home-based care.

STRATEGIES FOR ASSESSING COMPETENCIES IN PROFESSIONAL GEROPSYCHOLOGY

The Pikes Peak Geropsychology Knowledge and Skill Assessment Tool (Karel et al., 2010) tracks the development of attitudes, knowledge, and skills over time (see Appendix 1.2). In some formal training programs, mentors and trainees both complete the tool on a regular (e.g., annual) basis. Comparisons of ratings by trainers and trainees can be part of a process evaluation of the trainee and the program. Postlicensure practitioners can use this tool for self-assessment or to track the development of junior colleagues toward their own professional goals. Self-assessment guides the practitioner toward priorities for additional training, and if used over time, also tracks progress toward competency goals. With the growth of group practices and the integration of psychologists into other service delivery systems, psychologists may also find the tool to be useful in training colleagues who are new to geropsychological practice or new to practice with particular types of older adult clients or patients (e.g., chronically ill, seriously mentally ill, long-term-care residential).

STRATEGIES FOR ACHIEVING COMPETENCIES IN PROFESSIONAL GEROPSYCHOLOGY

The geropsychology competencies are intended to be aspirational (Knight et al., 2009), setting a standard for individuals to aspire to rather than one to be used as a minimal entry point. Thus, application of the competencies to entry-level psychologists can be detailed, using guidance available in Molinari (2012). A useful description of the use of competencies to guide self-assessment and development in licensed psychologists is offered by Karel, Knight, Duffy, Hinrichsen, and Zeiss (2010). They apply the competencies content to cases that are likely to be encountered by psychologists in a general practice setting, noting the competencies that may not be fully developed even in a licensed psychologist if she or he did not train to specialize in work with older adults. Of course, training opportunities are relevant to persons who have some training in geropsychology because even geropsychology experts will not have expertise in all domains of the competencies.

Formal training opportunities for postlicensure psychologists are limited. A full-year postdoctoral fellowship often is not attractive or realistic to a person with decades of work experience. Licensed psychologists are more likely to rely on continuing education workshops, webinars, or other distance learning strategies. Increasingly, such offerings are announced on e-mail lists of organizations invested in geropsychology training.

A particularly important strategy for professional development is membership in professional organizations that offer trainings, newsletters, and electronic mailing lists. Key organizations for geropsychologists are the Society of Clinical Geropsychology (n.d.), APA Division 20 (Division on Adult Development and Aging; n.d.), and Psychologists in Long-Term Care (n.d.). Regular perusal of the website of the APA Office on Aging (n.d.) also is useful because it serves as a repository of guidelines and resources. For example, that website offers immediate access to the APA Caregiver Briefcase, a rich resource for practitioners working with family caregivers. It also has available in an easy-to-download format handbooks related to capacity assessment, including one written specifically for psychologists (American Bar Association Commission on Law and Aging and American Psychological Association, 2008).

Self-guided reading is a common strategy professionals use to keep up on the literature. Bibliographies of recommended readings are usually offered by workshop presenters and may be found on the websites of organizations and handbooks in the field. The course syllabi posted on the website for APA Division 20 (n.d.) are also sources of excellent readings that are considered the standard in current graduate education.

Experiential learning needs to be part of the strategy of professionals seeking to expand their competency. Experiential learning is particularly critical for gaining skill in (a) helping clients access services in the senior network, (b) recognizing subtle signs of cognitive impairment, and (c) working with medical comorbidities. These areas may or may not be in the knowledge and skill base of psychologists, so they may be particularly hard to navigate clinically without some coaching.

Psychologists wishing to formalize their expertise in geropsychology will be interested in achieving board certification. Following the recognition of geropsychology as a specialty by the APA in 2010 (Molinari, 2011), a working group developed a board certification process. The American Board of Geropsychology (ABGERO) is, at the time of this writing, in the implementation phase of the formal affiliation process with the Specialty Board of the American Board of Professional Psychology. For additional information on the current status of ABGERO and procedures for applying for board certification, see ABGERO (n.d.) or the websites for the Council for Professional Training in Geropsychology (n.d.) and the APA Office on Aging (n.d.).

APPENDIX 1.1: ATTITUDE, KNOWLEDGE, AND SKILL COMPETENCIES FOR PRACTICE IN PROFESSIONAL GEROPSYCHOLOGY[1]

I. ATTITUDES

1. Psychologists are encouraged to work with older adults within their scope of competence and to seek consultation or make appropriate referrals when indicated.
2. Psychologists are encouraged to recognize how their attitudes and beliefs about aging and about older individuals may be relevant to their assessment and treatment of older adults and to seek consultation or further education about these issues when indicated.
3. Psychologists are encouraged to expand their awareness of how individual diversity in all of its manifestations (including gender, age, cohort, ethnicity, language, religion, socioeconomic status, sexual orientation, gender identity, disability status, and urban or rural residence) interacts with attitudes and beliefs about aging, to use this awareness to inform their assessment and treatment of older adults, and to seek consultation or further education when indicated.
4. Psychologists are encouraged to increase their knowledge, understanding, and skills with respect to working with older adults through continuing education, training, supervision, and consultation.

II. KNOWLEDGE BASE

A. Knowledge: General Knowledge About Adult Development, Aging, and the Older Adult Population

1. Theoretical models and research methodologies for understanding the processes of aging, including the life span developmental perspective, conceptions of positive or successful aging, and methodological issues in conducting or evaluating research on aging

---

[1]From "Attitude, Knowledge, and Skill Competencies for Practice in Professional Geropsychology," retrieved from http://www.copgtp.org. Copyright by the Council of Professional Geropsychology Training Programs. Reprinted with permission.

2. Demographics of aging, including where to obtain current knowledge on changes in population dynamics
3. Normal or "usual" aging, including the following:
   - Biological and health-related aspects of aging and mind–body interactions
   - Psychology of aging, including normative continuity and change in the domains of sensory processes, cognition, personality, and emotions
   - Social dynamics of the aging process, including issues such as work and retirement, friendships, roles, and family relationships
4. Awareness of diversity in the aging process, particularly how sociocultural factors such as gender, age, cohort, ethnicity, language, religion, socioeconomic status, sexual orientation, gender identity, disability status, and urban–rural residence may influence the experience and expression of health and of psychological problems in later life and how this knowledge may inform the assessment and treatment of older adults

B. Knowledge: Foundations of Clinical Practice With Older Adults

1. The neuroscience of aging, its applications to changes in cognition, and its implications for clinical interventions with older adults
2. Knowledge of the salience of functional changes in later adulthood, including resulting problems in daily living
3. Awareness of the concept of person–environment interaction and the implications of this concept for adaptation in late life
4. Psychopathology in middle and later adulthood, including differences in the prevalence, etiology, presentation, associated features, comorbidity, and course of mental disorders in older adults, as well as the health-related consequences of treated and untreated psychological disorders in late life
5. Knowledge of common acute, chronic, and terminal medical illnesses in late life

C. Knowledge: Foundations of Assessment of Older Adults

1. Theory and research informing psychological assessment of older adults, including the broad array of assessment domains,

methods, and instruments that are psychometrically suitable for assessing older adults

2. Issues in the limits of using assessment instruments created for younger persons with older adults without adequate standardization

3. Knowledge of contextual issues in the assessment of older adults, including the system or environment in which the elder functions, and the impact on assessment process and outcomes

D. Knowledge: Foundations of Intervention, Consultation, and Other Service Provision

1. Theory, research, and practice of various methods of intervention with older adults, including current research evidence about their efficacy and effectiveness as applied to diverse groups within the older adult population

2. Health, illness, and pharmacology as related to assessment and treatment of late-life mental health problems, including awareness of medical or medication factors that may affect treatment outcomes (e.g., illness, medication side effects, polypharmacy)

3. Issues pertaining to the provision of services in the specific settings in which older adults typically live or seek treatment

4. Knowledge of aging services in the local community (e.g., day care, transportation, residential) and how to refer clients to these services

5. Prevention and health promotion services and their relevance for middle-age and older adults at risk for mental disorders

6. Awareness of the broad array of potential clients (e.g., family members, other caregivers, health care professionals, and organizations) for psychological consultation and intervention and appropriate intervention strategies in these contexts

7. Models and methods of interdisciplinary collaboration, including an understanding of the varied components, roles, and contexts of interdisciplinary treatment of late-life mental disorders

8. Knowledge of ethical and legal standards related to psychological intervention with older adults and care systems, with particular attention to aging-specific issues of informed consent, confidentiality, substitute or end-of-life decision making and potential conflicts of interest, capacity and competency, and elder abuse and neglect

III. SKILL COMPETENCIES

A. Skills: Professional Geropsychology Functioning (Foundational Competencies)

1. Understand and apply ethical and legal standards, with particular attention to aging-specific issues, such as informed consent, confidentiality, capacity and competency, end-of-life decision making, and elder abuse and neglect.
2. Understand cultural and individual diversity as relevant to assessment, intervention, and consultation and apply to practice with diverse older adults.
3. Address complex biopsychosocial issues among many older adults by collaborating with other disciplines in multi- and interdisciplinary teams.
4. Practice self-reflection, self-assessment (e.g., self-awareness of ageist assumptions and biases, recognition of boundaries of competence and when and how to refer elsewhere).
5. Relate effectively and empathically with older adult clients, families, and other stakeholders in a range of professional roles and settings (e.g., senior center, hospital, long-term care).
6. Apply scientific knowledge to geropsychology practice and policy advocacy.
7. Practice appropriate documentation, billing, and reimbursement procedures for geropsychological services in compliance with state and federal laws and regulations (especially regarding Medicare and Medicaid services), including assessment and documentation of medical necessity.
8. Advocate for clients' needs and provide case management for needed services.

B. Skills: Assessment

1. Conduct clinical assessment leading to *Diagnostic and Statistical Manual of Mental Disorders* diagnoses and other clinically relevant problems, formulation of treatment plans, and, specifically, differential diagnosis (common problems and issues include but are not limited to depression, anxiety, grief, delirium, dementia, and medication effects, and physical disorders and their effects on functioning).
2. Use psychometrically sound screening instruments for cognition, psychopathology, and personality to inform treatment planning.

3. Refer for neuropsychological, neurological, psychiatric, medical or other evaluations as indicated.
4. Use cognitive assessments and/or neuropsychological reports to clarify clinical issues and inform treatment planning.
5. Evaluate decision-making and functional capacities (e.g., for managing finances, independent living, driving, making health care decisions).
6. Assess risk (e.g., suicidality, self-neglect, elder abuse).
7. Adapt instruments and tailor assessments to accommodate older adults' specific characteristics and contexts.
8. Communicate assessment results to various stakeholders with relevant, practical, and clearly understandable recommendations, with appropriate consideration for confidentiality issues.

C. Skills: Intervention

1. Apply individual, group, and family interventions to older adults using appropriate modifications to accommodate distinctive bio-psychosocial functioning of older adults and distinct therapeutic relationship characteristics.
2. Use available evidence-based treatments for older adults.
3. Develop psychotherapeutic interventions based on empirical literature, theory, and clinical judgment when insufficient efficacy research is available on older adults.
4. Be proficient in using commonly applied late-life interventions such as those focusing on life review, grief, end-of-life care, and caregiving.
5. Use interventions to enhance the health of diverse elderly persons (e.g., chronic health problems, healthy aging, cognitive fitness).
6. Demonstrate ability to intervene in settings where older adults and their family members are often seen (e.g., health services, housing, community programs) with a range of strategies including those targeted at the individual, family, environment, and system.

D. Skills: Consultation/Training

1. Consult to families, professionals, programs, health care facilities, legal systems, and other agencies and organizations that serve older adults.
2. Provide training on geropsychological issues (e.g., in-services, workshops, community education) to different disciplines.

3. Participate in interprofessional teams that serve older adults.
4. Communicate psychological conceptualizations to medical and other professionals in a concise and useful manner.
5. Implement strategies for systems analysis and change in organizations and facilities that serve older adults.
6. Design and participate in different models of aging services delivery (e.g., integrated care).
7. Collaborate and coordinate with other agencies and professionals that serve older adults.
8. Recognize and negotiate multiple roles in older adult consultation settings.

E. Skills: Delivery of Services in Different Settings

Delivery of services in two or more different settings, including the following:

1. Outpatient mental health services
2. Outpatient primary care or medical settings
3. Inpatient medical service
4. Inpatient psychiatric service
5. Long-term care settings including nursing homes, assisted living facilities, home care, day programs
6. Rehabilitation settings
7. Hospice
8. Community-based programs
9. Forensic settings
10. Home-delivered psychological services
11. Research settings

APPENDIX 1.2: PIKES PEAK MODEL COMPETENCIES TOOL[2]

PIKES PEAK GEROPSYCHOLOGY KNOWLEDGE AND SKILL ASSESSMENT TOOL

Council of Professional Geropsychology Training Programs
Version 1.1 © 2008, Version 1.2 © 2011, Version 1.3 © 2012

PURPOSE

This evaluation tool is for learners who are working to develop knowledge and skills for providing optimal care to older adults, their families, and related care systems. Psychology trainees, their supervisors, and practicing psychologists may use this tool to evaluate progress in developing geropsychology competencies and to help define ongoing learning goals and training needs.

PIKES PEAK COMPETENCIES

Competencies for professional geropsychology practice were delineated during the 2006 National Conference on Training in Professional Geropsychology. Taken together, the competencies are aspirational, rather than "required" of any particular psychologist. Even the most accomplished geropsychologist will have relative strengths and weaknesses across the spectrum of competencies for geropsychology. The conference produced the Pikes Peak Model for Geropsychology Training (Knight et al., 2008) and created the Council of Professional Geropsychology Training Programs (CoPGTP, see http://www.copgtp.org/). CoPGTP developed this competency evaluation tool for learners and supervisors to have a measure by which to gauge

---

[2]From "Pikes Peak Geropsychology Knowledge and Skill Assessment Tool," retrieved from http://www.copgtp.org. Copyright 2012 by the Council of Professional Geropsychology Training Programs. Reprinted with permission.

competence in serving older adults.[3] For the purposes of this evaluation tool, each Pikes Peak geropsychology knowledge and skill competency is specified by behaviorally descriptive items, and can be rated along a continuum from Novice to Expert. Some redundancy is inherent in this measure. The intent is to evaluate both the learner's knowledge base and skill set separately for the same domains, as the awareness of information and ability or experience in applying it may differ.

GEROPSYCHOLOGY PRACTICE

Geropsychologists provide assessment, intervention, consultation, and other professional services across a wide range of medical, mental health, residential, community, and other care settings with a population of demographically and socioculturally diverse older adults. The Pikes Peak competencies are applicable across varied geriatric care settings and populations. It is recognized also that each work area or training setting may call for the development of particular competencies, not all of which may be addressed in this document. Both the APA *Guidelines for Psychological Practice With Older Adults* (APA, 2014) and the Pikes Peak Model highlight core attitudes for practice with older adults. Although this tool does not evaluate attitudes explicitly, the knowledge and skill competencies reflect core geropsychology practice attitudes, including recognition of scope of competence, self-awareness of attitudes and beliefs about aging and older adults, appreciation of diversity among older adults, and commitment to continuing education.

USING THE COMPETENCY EVALUATION TOOL

This tool is intended to be used both by supervisors to assess trainees and by psychologists to assess their own knowledge and skills. Supervisors in geropsychology training programs may choose to evaluate the domains relevant to the goals of their program. Evaluation should include the learner's perspective (self-assessment), observation of the learner's work (e.g., direct observation, audiotape, videotape, co-therapy), as well as regular supervision involving case discussion. Psychologists and trainees conducting self-assessments can use the tool to evaluate their training and supervision needs in each area. The tool also can gauge a learner's progress over time.

---

[3]Development of this evaluation tool was informed by several important previous efforts, including the APA policies on multicultural and evidence-based practice, extensive work on the assessment of competencies for professional psychology practice, competencies for geriatric and palliative care, and evaluation tools that have been used by geropsychology internship and fellowship programs. An abbreviated reference list follows.

The learner can be rated on each Pikes Peak knowledge domain and skill competency as Novice (N), Intermediate (I), Advanced (A), Proficient (P), or Expert (E), as described below. Each Pikes Peak competency (highlighted in light gray in the chart below) is delineated by several specifiers (indicated by letters *a*, *b*, *c*, etc., in the chart). The specifiers are designed to help define the knowledge domain or skill competency and **do not need to be rated separately**. However, the specifiers can be rated individually if that level of assessment is desired.

RATING SCALE ANCHORS

This rating scale assumes that professional competence is developed over time, as learners develop knowledge and skills with ongoing education, training, and supervision. The anchors, then, reflect developmental levels of competence, from Novice through Expert. The scale is adapted from previous efforts, as summarized by Hatcher and Lassiter (2007). Because the scale reflects development of competence, the same scale can be used at different levels of training. For example, graduate practica students would be expected to perform at Novice through Advanced levels, while postdoctoral fellows in geropsychology would be expected to perform from Intermediate to Proficient levels. Development of knowledge and skills may differ significantly across domains, depending upon previous training experiences.

To illustrate use of the scale, we provide a brief vignette and how an individual at each level might approach the case.

> **Vignette:** *A 78-year-old Irish-American man is referred to the mental health clinic by his primary care physician because his daughter-in-law complained that, in recent months, he has become depressed and forgetful and is no longer involved in his hobbies. He has several chronic medical problems including mild diabetes and hypertension. His Korean American wife of 52 years is angry that he is not completing his household chores. His three adult children have varied levels of involvement in his life, with one daughter and one son living nearby. He comes to the clinic for an initial evaluation.*

Novice (N): Possesses entry-level skills; needs intensive supervision

Novices have limited knowledge and understanding of case conceptualization and intervention skills, and the processes and techniques of implementing them. Novices do not yet recognize consistent patterns of behavior relevant for diagnosis and care planning and do not differentiate well between important and unimportant details.

Example: The learner is able to identify salient symptoms, but does not appreciate possible contributions of medical, neurological, and family system factors to the older adult's presentation, and does not know how to formulate differential diagnosis questions.

Intermediate (I): Has a background of some exposure and experience; ongoing supervision is needed

Experience has been gained through practice, supervision, and instruction. The learner is able to recognize important recurring issues and select appropriate strategies. Generalization of skills is limited and support is needed to guide performance.

Example: The learner recognizes multiple possible contributions to the older adult's presentation, is able to collect history from the patient (and his daughter-in-law, with his permission), administer depression and cognitive screening tools, and consult with supervisor to discuss possible implications and to plan further evaluation. Learner may not appreciate complex, late-life family and cultural systems issues affecting patient's coping.

Advanced (A): Has solid experience, handles typical situations well; requires supervision for unusual or complex situations

Knowledge of the competency domain is more integrated, including application of appropriate research literature. The learner is more fluent in the ability to recognize patterns and select appropriate strategies to guide diagnosis and treatment

Example: The learner is able to integrate multiple sources of information (e.g., behavioral observation, cognitive testing data, medical records, collateral reports) and complex history (medical, psychiatric, family, occupational, and cultural context) to rule out possibility of early dementia plus depression, and make recommendations to the primary care provider and family about further assessment and treatment options. Learner consults with supervisor about local resources for older adults, and how best to handle issues around wife's difficulty coping with patient's changes, related marital conflict, family dynamics, culture, and treatment planning.

Proficient (P): Functions autonomously, knows limits of ability; seeks supervision or consultation as needed

Proficiency is demonstrated in perceiving situations as wholes and not only summations of parts, including an appreciation of longer term implications of current situation. The psychologist has a perspective on which of the many existing attributes and aspects in the present situation are important ones, and has developed a nuanced understanding of the clinical situation.

Example: Learner is able to integrate information, as above, collaborate with family and medical (e.g., psychiatrist, neurologist) and social service providers for ongoing assessment and intervention for the patient and family (e.g., psychoeducation, couple's therapy, explore community support options). Learner functions as a full member of an interdisciplinary team to address the biopsychosocial needs of the client and his family, and is able to assume a leadership role.

Expert (E): Serves as resource or consultant to others, is recognized as having expertise

With significant background of experience, the geropsychologist is able to focus in on the essentials of the problem quickly and efficiently. Analytical problem solving is used to consider unfamiliar situations, or when initial impressions do not bear out.

Example: Learner is frequently contacted by other psychologists in her community to provide consultation regarding care of older adults with dementia. Learner is able to use the above case as a teaching example for the need to provide a thorough biopsychosocial assessment in geriatric care, to implement an interdisciplinary team plan, and to be knowledgeable about geriatric resources in the community.

Note. Ratings are only needed where the anchors are provided (indicated by Arabic numbers 1, 2, 3, etc. in the chart). Specifiers (indicated by letters a, b, c, etc. in the chart) are designed to help define the knowledge domain or skill competency and do not need to be rated separately, unless that level of assessment is desired.

I. General Knowledge About Adult Development, Aging, and the Older Adult Population	
A. The psychologist/trainee has <u>KNOWLEDGE OF</u>:	
1. Models of Aging	**N I A P E**
a. Development as a lifelong process encompassing early to late life, and encompassing both gains and losses over the life span	
b. Different theories of late-life development and adaptation	
c. Biopsychosocial perspective for understanding an individual's physical and psychological development within the sociocultural context	
d. Concept of, and variables associated with, positive or successful aging	
e. Relevant research on adult development and aging, including methodological considerations in cross-sectional and longitudinal research.	
2. Demographics	**N I A P E**
a. Demographic trends of the aging population, including gender, racial, ethnic, and socioeconomic heterogeneity	

	NIAPE
b. Resources to remain updated on the demographics of aging, including internet sites for: U.S. Census, Centers for Disease Control and Prevention, Social Security Administration, Bureau of Labor Statistics, National Institutes of Health, World Health Organization.	
3. Normal Aging—Biological, Psychological, Social Aspects	**N I A P E**
a. Physical changes in later life	
b. Normal aging as distinct from disease, regarding both physical and mental health	
c. Interactions among physical changes, health behaviors, stress, personality, and mental health in older adults	
d. Aging-related changes in sensory processes including vision, hearing, touch, taste, and smell	
e. Aging-related changes in sexual functioning	
f. Aging-related changes in cognitive processes, including attention, memory, executive functioning, language, and intellectual functions	
g. Aging-related changes in personality	
h. Aging-related changes in emotional expression and coping mechanisms	
i. Factors that influence vocational satisfaction, job performance, leisure activities, retirement satisfaction, and volunteer participation	
j. Family dynamics and role changes in aging families	
k. Changing social networks in late life, and value of close friendships in later life	
4. Diversity in Aging Experience	**N I A P E**
a. The diversity of the older adult population, and that age alone is a poor predictor of an individual's functioning	
b. The unique experience of each individual—based on demographic, sociocultural, and life experiences—and that multiple factors interact over the life span to influence an older individual's patterns of behavior	
c. Historical influences affecting particular cohorts	

II. Foundations of Professional Geropsychology Practice	
A. Knowledge Base—The psychologist/trainee has **<u>KNOWLEDGE OF</u>:**	
1. Neuroscience of Aging	**N I A P E**
a. The parameters of cognitive changes in normal aging, including their basis in age-related changes in the brain	
b. Factors that influence levels of cognitive performance in older adults (e.g., genetics, socioeconomic status, cohort effects, health status, mood, medications/substances)	
c. Common types of dementia in terms of onset, etiology, risk factors, clinical course, associated behavioral features, and medical management of these disorders	
d. Characteristics and causes of mild cognitive impairment and reversible cognitive impairment, including delirium, and the pathway to their management or reversal	
e. Clinical interventions which target behavioral features and psychological problems in individuals with cognitive disorders and their caregivers	
2. Functional Changes	**N I A P E**
a. Relationships between age, environment, and functional level	
b. Definition and assessment of Activities of Daily Living (ADLs) and Instrumental Activities of Daily Living (IADLs)	
c. Relationship between functional abilities and decisions older adults make with regard to employment, healthcare, relationships, lifestyle and leisure activities, and living environment	
d. Relationship between functional ability and psychopathology in older adults, including how functional ability of older persons affects family members	
e. Strategies commonly used by older adults to cope with functional limitations	
3. Person–Environment Interaction and **Adaptation**	**N I A P E**
a. Interaction of an elder's abilities and needs with the demands and opportunities provided by various living and treatment environments (e.g., private homes, assisted living facilitates, nursing facilities)	

	N I A P E
b. Impact of aging stereotypes on an older individual's functional status and self-efficacy	
c. Importance and complexities around issues of maintaining optimal independence and optimal safety, particularly when medical conditions and cognitive disorders impair the elder's functioning	
d. Ethical and legal issues which arise in the context of markedly impaired functional status and decision making capacity	
e. Situations and signs that suggest risk for abuse and neglect	
4. Psychopathology	**N I A P E**
a. Biopsychosocial etiological models, applied within a life span developmental and cohort relevant context, for major psychological disorders affecting older adults	
b. Differential presentation, associated features, age of onset, and course of common psychological disorders and syndromes in older adults (e.g., anxiety, depression, dementia, etc.)	
c. Variations in presentations of psychopathology in later life due to cohort, cognitive, medical and pharmacological issues, including lifelong mental illness and late onset mental illness	
d. Under-recognized aspects of psychopathology in late life which affect functional impairment and safety (e.g., suicide risk, substance use, complicated grief)	
e. Interaction of common mental illnesses with the more common medical illnesses and medications and implications involved for assessment and treatment	
f. Psychosocial, psychotherapeutic, and psychopharmacological approaches to treating psychological disorders in older adults, as well as the health-related consequences of not treating and side effects of the possible treatments	
5. Medical Illness	**N I A P E**
a. Common medical and neurological problems (e.g., cardio- and cerebro-vascular disorders), syndromes (e.g., falls, incontinence), and substances or medications (e.g., alcohol, benzodiazepines, narcotics, over-the-counter remedies) associated with psychopathology in older adults	

b. Multiple pathways of interaction between medical illness and psychopathology in late life	
c. Common medical tests (e.g., thyroid function, urinalysis, CT/MRI) relevant to differentiating medical and psychological illness in late life	
d. Relationships between chronic pain, functioning, and mental health in older adults (e.g., relationship of depression to pain)	
6. End-of-Life Issues	**N I A P E**
a. Physical, cognitive, emotional, and spiritual components of advanced illness and the dying process	
b. Diversity in ethnic, cultural, and spiritual beliefs and rituals involved in death and the dying process	
c. Models of hospice and palliative care	
d. Impact of advanced illness, caregiving, dying and death on family members	
e. Differences between normal grief reactions and complicated grief	
B. Professional Geropsychology Functioning—Foundational SKILLS—The psychologist/trainee is _ABLE TO_:	
1. Apply Ethical and Legal Standards by Identifying, Analyzing, and Addressing	**N I A P E**
Identify complex ethical and legal issues that arise in the care of older adults, analyze them accurately, and proactively address them, including:	
a. Tension between sometimes competing goals of promoting autonomy and protecting safety of at-risk older adults	
b. Decision-making capacity and strategies for optimizing older adults' participation in informed consent regarding a wide range of medical, residential, financial, and other life decisions	
c. Surrogate decision-making as indicated regarding a wide range of medical, residential, financial, end-of-life, and other life decisions	
d. State and organizational laws and policies covering elder abuse, advance directives, conservatorship, guardianship, multiple relationships, and confidentiality	

2. Address Cultural and Individual Diversity With Older Adults, Families, Communities, and Systems/Providers by Being Able to	N I A P E
a. Recognize gender, age, cohort, ethnic/racial, cultural, linguistic, socioeconomic, religious, disability, sexual orientation, gender identity, and urban/rural residence variations in the aging process	
b. Articulate integrative conceptualizations of multiple aspects of diversity influencing older clients, psychologists, and systems of care	
c. Adapt professional behavior in a culturally sensitive manner, as appropriate to the needs of the older client	
d. Work effectively with diverse providers, staff, and students in care settings serving older adults	
e. Demonstrate self-awareness and ability to recognize differences between the clinician's and the patient's values, attitudes, assumptions, hopes and fears related to aging, caregiving, illness, disability, social supports, medical care, dying, grief	
f. Initiate consultation with appropriate sources as needed to address specific diversity issues	
3. Recognize Importance of Teams	N I A P E
a. Understand the theory and science of geriatric team building	
b. Value the role that other providers play in the assessment and treatment of older clients	
c. Demonstrate awareness, appreciation, and respect for team experiences, values, and discipline-specific conceptual models	
d. Understand the importance of teamwork in geriatric settings to address the varied biopsychosocial needs of older adults	
4. Practice Self-Reflection	N I A P E
a. Demonstrate awareness of personal biases, assumptions, stereotypes, and potential discomfort in working with older adults, particularly those of backgrounds divergent from the psychologist	

	N I A P E
b. Monitor internal thoughts and feelings that may influence professional behavior, and adjust behavior accordingly in order to focus on needs of the patient, family, and treatment team	
c. Demonstrate accurate self-evaluation of knowledge and skill competencies related to work with diverse older adults, including those with particular diagnoses, or in particular care settings	
d. Initiate consultation with or referral to appropriate providers when uncertain about one's own competence	
e. Seek continuing education, training, supervision, and consultation to enhance geropsychology competencies related to practice	
5. Relate Effectively and Empathically	**N I A P E**
a. Use rapport and empathy in verbal and nonverbal behaviors to facilitate interactions with older adults, families, and care teams	
b. Form effective working alliance with wide range of older clients, families, colleagues, and other stakeholders	
c. Communicate new knowledge to patients and families, adjusting language and complexity of concepts based on the patient and family's level of sensory and cognitive capabilities, educational background, knowledge, values, and developmental stage	
d. Demonstrate awareness, appreciation, and respect for older patient, family, and team experiences, values, and conceptual models	
e. Demonstrate appreciation of client and organizational strengths, as well as deficits and challenges, and capitalize on strengths in planning interventions	
f. Tolerate and understand interpersonal conflict and differences within or between older patients, families, and team members, and negotiate conflict effectively	
6. Apply Scientific Knowledge	**N I A P E**
a. Demonstrate awareness of scientific knowledge base in adult development and aging; biomedical, psychological, and social gerontology; and geriatric health and mental health care; incorporate this knowledge into geriatric health and mental health practice	

b. Apply review of available scientific literature to case conceptualization, treatment planning, and intervention	
c. Acknowledge strengths and limitations of knowledge base in application to individual case	
d. Demonstrate ability to cite scientific evidence on aging to support professional activities in academic, clinical and policy settings	
7. Practice Appropriate Business of Geropsychology	**N I A P E**
a. Demonstrate awareness of Medicare, Medicaid, and other insurance coverage for diagnostic conditions and health and mental health care services	
b. Demonstrate appropriate diagnostic and procedure coding for psychological services rendered	
c. Demonstrate medical record documentation that is consistent with Medicare, Medicaid, HIPAA, and other federal, state, or local or organizational regulations, including appropriate documentation of medical necessity for services	
d. Remain updated on policy and regulatory changes that affect practice, such as through professional newsletters and e-mail forums	
e. Demonstrate understanding of quality indicators for the care of older adults with mental disorders	
8. Advocate and Provide Care Coordination	**N I A P E**
a. Demonstrate awareness of potential individual and psychosocial barriers to the ability of older adults to access and utilize health, mental health, or community services	
b. Collaborate with patients, families, and other organizational and community providers to improve older adults' access to needed health care, residential, transportation, social, or community services	
c. Advocate for clients' needs in interdisciplinary and organizational environments when appropriate	

III. Assessment	
A. Knowledge Base—The psychologist/trainee has <u>KNOWLEDGE OF</u>:	
1. Geropsychology Assessment Methods	**N I A P E**
a. Current research and literature relevant to understanding theory and current trends in geropsychology assessment	
b. Assessment measures or techniques which have been developed, normed, validated and determined to be psychometrically suitable for use with older adults	
c. Importance of a comprehensive interdisciplinary assessment approach (e.g., including other health professionals' evaluations of medical or social issues)	
d. Multimethod approach to assessing older adults (including cognitive, psychological, personality, and behavioral assessments, drawn from self-report, interviews, and observational methods)	
e. Importance of integrating collateral information from family, friends, and caregivers, with appropriate consent, especially when cognitive impairment is suspected	
f. Need for baseline and repeated-measures assessments in order to understand complex diagnostic problems	
g. Assessment of domains unique to older adults (e.g., potential elder abuse)	
2. Limitations of Assessment Methods	**N I A P E**
a. Criterion and age requirements, as well as specific standard normative data, for testing instruments	
b. Limitations of testing instruments, including those validated in older samples, for assessing diverse older adults	
3. Contextual Issues in Geropsychology Assessment	**N I A P E**
a. The range of potential individual factors that may affect assessment performance (e.g., medications, substance use, medical conditions, cultural, educational, language background)	
b. The potential impact of the assessment environment on test performance (e.g., noise, lighting, distractions)	
c. The older person's environmental context and resources in deriving recommendations from assessment data	

B. SKILLS—The psychologist/trainee is <u>ABLE TO</u>:	
1. Conduct Clinical Assessment and Differential Diagnosis	**N I A P E**
a. Distinguish between signs of normal aging versus pathology in making diagnoses	
b. Consider base rates, risk factors, and distinct symptom presentations of psychological disorders in older adults when making diagnoses	
c. Conduct differential diagnosis (e.g., dementia versus depression), including consideration of comorbid medical issues that may influence an older adult's presentation	
d. Identify subsyndromal disorders and implications for treatment	
e. Assess older adult's motivation for treatment	
f. Utilize biopsychosocial case conceptualization based on clinical evaluation to inform initial treatment plan or recommendations	
2. Utilize Screening Instruments	**N I A P E**
a. Utilize screening tools for mood, cognition, substance use, personality, and other clinical issues to guide and inform comprehensive assessment	
b. Evaluate age, educational, and cultural appropriateness of assessment instruments	
c. Consider reliability and validity data in using standardized instruments with older adults	
d. Assess older adult's ability to provide informed consent for psychological evaluation	
e. Recognize sensory impairments and makes environmental modifications accordingly	
f. Consider impact of medical conditions and medications on test performance	
g. Make specific and appropriate recommendations, based on testing results, to inform treatment planning	
3. Refer for Other Evaluations as Indicated	**N I A P E**
a. Acknowledge personal level of expertise regarding geriatric assessment and know when to refer or consult with other health care professionals	

b. Utilize screening data to inform need for more comprehensive, multidisciplinary assessment	
c. Recognize when a medical evaluation is indicated to rule out underlying medical or pharmacological causes of presenting symptoms	
4. Utilize Cognitive Assessments	**N I A P E**
a. Integrate knowledge of normal and pathological aging, including age-related changes in cognitive abilities, into geropsychological evaluations	
b. Interpret meaning and implications of cognitive testing data or reports for case conceptualization	
c. Demonstrate ability to translate cognitive testing results into practical conclusions and recommendations for patients, families, and other care providers	
5. Evaluate Decision-Making and Functional Capacity	**N I A P E**
a. Evaluate older adults' understanding, appreciation, reasoning, and choice abilities with regards to capacity for decision making	
b. Utilize clinically specific assessment tools designed to aid evaluation of decision-making and other functional capacities	
c. Integrate testing results with information from clinical interview with older adult and collateral sources, including behavioral observations and interviews with family members, to formulate impressions and recommendations	
d. Collaborate with professionals from other disciplines to assess specific functional capacities (e.g., independent living, driving)	
e. Appreciate legal and clinical contexts of capacity/competence evaluations (e.g., need for guardianship, loss of right to drive)	
6. Assess Risk	**N I A P E**
a. Identify risk factors for harm to self or others	
b. Screen and comprehensively assesses suicide risk	
c. Screen and assesses capacity for self-care including ADLs and IADLs	

d. Screen and assesses risk of elder abuse in emotional, physical, sexual, financial, and neglect domains	
7. Communicate Assessment Results and Recommendations	**N I A P E**
a. Communicate results within the confines of federal, state, local, and institutional privacy and confidentiality rules and regulations	
b. Translate assessment results into practical recommendations for patient, family, and team, providing written recommendations and relevant psychoeducational materials understandable to stakeholders	
c. Provide recommendations to other providers to assure that treatment plans are informed by assessment results	
IV. Intervention	
A. Knowledge—The psychologist/trainee has <u>KNOWLEDGE OF</u>:	
1. Theory, Research, and Practice	**N I A P E**
a. Broad research findings regarding the effectiveness of psychological interventions with older adults (e.g., application of behavioral, cognitive, interpersonal, psychodynamic, family, environmental, psychoeducational, group interventions)	
b. Specialized interventions in working with older adults and how they evolve from and are consistent with theory in life span development (e.g., reminiscence therapy, validation techniques, behavioral interventions for disruptive behavior)	
c. Modifications of therapeutic techniques to address common aging changes (e.g., sensory difficulties, cognitive impairment), care setting (e.g., community, hospital, nursing home), education, and cultural background	
2. Health, Illness, and Pharmacology	**N I A P E**
a. The complexity and interplay of common late-life medical problems, sensory changes and their impact on treatment approaches	

b. The possible impact of medications and procedures for medical and psychiatric problems, including detrimental side effects, on symptom presentation, mental status, and treatment effectiveness in older adults	
c. The frequent comorbidity between chronic medical and psychiatric problems, and need to address both medical and mental health issues	
d. The importance of setting realistic treatment goals (neither too high nor too low) for older adults with severe, chronic medical and psychiatric problems (e.g., remission of symptoms or maintenance of current functioning rather than cure)	
3. Specific Settings	**N I A P E**
a. The varied preferences older adults have in discussing emotional problems with family, primary care providers, spiritual advisors and, thus, the importance of allying with others, with appropriate consent, to assure proper psychological care is rendered	
b. The salience and presentation of ethical issues when employing interventions across varied care settings (e.g., confidentiality in context of team treatment planning; privacy constraints in institutional settings)	
c. Adaptations of interventions appropriate to particular settings (e.g., focus on staff education and behavioral, environmental interventions in long-term care settings)	
4. Aging Services	**N I A P E**
a. Specific referral sources including facilities (e.g., day care, residential), transportation, legal/safety (e.g., protective services), health, multicultural, caregiver, and other support services	
b. Referral processes and procedures to local community resources (e.g., via phone, Internet)	
c. Follow-up mechanism(s) regarding referrals	
5. Ethical and Legal Standards	**N I A P E**
a. Informed consent procedures for services to older adults, and challenges to some older adults' capacity to provide informed consent	

b. Indications for and role of surrogate decision makers in health and mental health treatment of older adults	
c. Older client's right to confidentiality and to be informed of limits of confidentiality	
d. State and organizational laws and policies covering elder abuse, advance directives, conservatorship, guardianship, restraints, multiple relationships, and confidentiality	

B. SKILLS—The psychologist/trainee is **ABLE TO:**

1. Apply Individual, Group, and Family Interventions	**N I A P E**
a. Prioritize treatment goals as appropriate, taking into account multiple problem areas	
b. Integrate relevant treatment modalities	
c. Modify evidence-based and clinically informed intervention strategies to accommodate chronic and acute medical problems, sensory impairments, mobility limitations, cognitive abilities, generational and cultural factors, late-life developmental issues and possible client-therapist age differences	
d. Provide psychoeducation as needed to help the older adult client understand the therapeutic process	
2. Base Interventions on Empirical Research, Theory, and Clinical Judgment	**N I A P E**
a. Articulate theoretical case conceptualization and empirical support guiding choice of intervention strategies	
b. Describe the integration or adaptation of various strategies to meet the needs of particular older clients	
c. Measure the effectiveness of intervention	
d. Make appropriate adjustments to treatment based on client response	
3. Use Available Evidence-Based Treatments for Older Adults	**N I A P E**
a. Choose evidence-based treatment for older adult clients based on diagnosis and other relevant client characteristics	
b. Choose and implement intervention strategies based on available evidence for effectiveness with older adults	

c. Measure the effectiveness of intervention	
d. Make appropriate adjustments to treatment based on client response	
4. Use Late-Life Interventions—Provide Effective, Evidence-based Interventions for Particular Issues Affecting Older Adults, including	N I A P E
a. For older adults with dementia (and other disabling illnesses) and their family caregivers	
b. For patients and families facing advanced illness, dying, and death	
c. For adjustment difficulties secondary to bereavement	
d. Inclusion of reminiscence and life review into psychotherapeutic interventions	
e. Psychoeducation for patients and families regarding normal aging and a range of medical and mental health concerns	
f. Group interventions for a range of aging-related health, mental health, and adjustment concerns	
g. For older adults adjusting to age-related changes in relationships and sexuality	
5. Use Health-Enhancing Interventions	N I A P E
a. Determine which aspects of physical, mental, and behavioral health can be improved in older clients via available psychological interventions	
b. Prioritize health issues to be addressed when multiple targets are possible	
c. Effectively intervene regarding health issues as part of overall mental health treatment plan, recognizing close link between medical and mental health and related disability in older adults	
d. Monitor impact of intervention on health behaviors and evaluates outcomes	
6. Intervene Across Settings	N I A P E
a. Intervene in common geriatric settings (e.g., home, community centers, nursing homes, assisted living facilities, retirement communities, medical clinics, medical and psychiatric hospitals)	

b. Intervene at the level appropriate to older adult client's needs, ranging from individual to family, systemic, and environmental contexts	
c. Modify interventions to adapt to the setting's particular environmental and social characteristics	

V. Consultation

A. Knowledge Base—The psychologist/trainee has KNOWLEDGE OF:

1. Prevention and Health Promotion	N I A P E
a. Incidence and prevalence rates of health problems in the older adult population	
b. How to partner with family and local community resources for health promotion	
c. Strategies for community-based training/education for promoting preventive interventions	

2. Diverse Clientele and Contexts	N I A P E
a. Multiple levels of geropsychological intervention/consultation, including individuals, families, healthcare professionals, organizations, and community leaders	
b. Systems-based consultative and intervention models and their use with appropriate modifications in different geriatric settings	
c. Strategies and methods for collaboration to address individual- and organizational-based needs	

3. Interdisciplinary Collaboration	N I A P E
a. The distinction between types of treatment teams (e.g., multidisciplinary and interdisciplinary)	
b. The roles, and potential contributions, of a wide range of healthcare professionals in the assessment and treatment of older adult with mental disorders	
c. How team composition and functioning may differ across settings of care	

B. SKILLS—The psychologist/trainee is ABLE TO:

1. Provide Geropsychological Consultation	N I A P E
a. Recognize situations in which geropsychological consultation is appropriate	

	N I A P E
b. Demonstrate ability to clarify and refine a referral question	
c. Demonstrate ability to gather information necessary to answer referral question	
d. Advocate for quality care for older adults with their families, professionals, programs, health care facilities, legal systems, and other agencies or organizations	
2. Provide Training	**N I A P E**
a. Assess learning needs of trainees related to varying levels of training and amount of experience within and across disciplines	
b. Define learning goals and objectives as a basis for developing educational sessions	
c. Provide clear, concise education that is appropriate for the level and learning needs of the trainees	
3. Participate in Interprofessional Teams	**N I A P E**
a. Work with professionals in other disciplines to incorporate geropsychological information into team treatment planning and implementation	
b. Communicate psychological conceptualizations clearly and respectfully to other providers	
c. Appreciate and integrate feedback from interdisciplinary team members into case conceptualizations	
d. Work to build consensus on treatment plans and goals of care, to invite various perspectives, and to negotiate conflict constructively	
e. Demonstrate ability to work with diverse team structures (e.g., hierarchical, lateral, virtual) and team members (e.g., including the ethics board, chaplains, and families in palliative care teams)	
4. Communicate Geropsychological Conceptualizations	**N I A P E**
a. Provide clear and concise written communication of geropsychological conceptualizations and recommendations	

b. Provide clear and concise oral communication of geropsychological conceptualizations and recommendations	
c. Uses appropriate language and level of detail for the target audience of the communication	
5. Implement Organizational Change	**N I A P E**
a. Conduct needs assessment for service delivery within the setting or program that serves older adults	
b. Develop policies and procedures for service delivery that involve all appropriate disciplines and staff members	
c. Evaluate effectiveness of service delivery model or program	
6. Participate in a Variety of Models of Aging Services Delivery	**N I A P E**
a. Differentiate goals and models of care in long-term, rehabilitation, acute, primary, home, assisted living, hospice, and other care settings	
b. Appreciate a variety of models of geriatric mental health care, including integrated mental health services in primary care, specialty consultation, and home- or community-based services	
c. Demonstrate awareness of strengths and constraints of various care models	
d. Demonstrate flexibility in professional roles to adapt to the realities of work in a variety of aging or healthcare delivery systems	
7. Collaborate and Coordinate With Other Agencies and Professionals	**N I A P E**
a. Work with team members to create smooth and efficient transitions across health care settings for older adults and their families	
b. Demonstrate respect for confidentiality and informed consent, as well as continuity of care, in coordinating with family members, other professionals, and agencies regarding care of an older client	
c. Establish working relationships with local and national agencies and organizations, such as Elder Services, Alzheimer's Association, and Hospice	

8. Recognize and Negotiate Multiple Roles	N I A P E
a. Identify the client and explicate the expectations of the relationship at the outset of the consultation	
b. Advocate on behalf of the well-being of older adults within each professional role, including when the individual or group of older adults is not the direct client	
c. Discuss potential conflicts of interest with colleagues and teams as indicated	
d. Discuss financial arrangements with all stakeholders	

SUMMARY

It may help learners and/or supervisors to summarize the geropsychology knowledge and skill strengths, and areas for growth, based on this assessment. Areas for growth may then be linked to further goals for education and training.

Strengths: Knowledge and skill domains in which the learner feels most confident and competent in geropsychology practice

Areas for Growth: Knowledge and skill domains in which the learner wishes to develop further competency

Education and Training Goals (within a practicum, internship rotation, fellowship, or post-licensure program of self-study)

APPENDIX 1.2 REFERENCES

American Psychological Association. (2003). Guidelines on multicultural education, training, research, practice, and organizational change for psychologists. *American Psychologist, 58,* 377–402.

American Psychological Association. (2004). Guidelines for psychological practice with older adults. *American Psychologist, 59,* 236–260.

American Psychological Association. (2006). *APA taskforce on the assessment of competence in professional psychology: Final report.* Washington, DC: Author.

APA Board of Educational Affairs and Council of Chairs of Training Councils. (2007). *Assessment of Competency Benchmarks Workgroup: A developmental model for the defining and measuring competence in professional psychology.* Retrieved from http://www.ccptp.org/2007-conference-resources.

APA Presidential Task Force on Evidence-Based Practice. (2006). Evidence-based practice in psychology. *American Psychologist, 61,* 271–285.

Hatcher, R. L. & Lassiter, K. D. (2007). Initial training in professional psychology: The practicum competencies outline. *Training and Education in Professional Psychology, 1,* 49–63.

Kaslow, N. J., Rubin, N. J., Bebeau, M. J., Leigh, I. W., Lichtenberg, J. W., Nelson, P. D., . . . Smith, I. L. (2007). Guiding principles and recommendations for the assessment of competence. *Professional Psychology: Research and Practice, 38,* 441.

Knight, B. G., Karel, M. J., Hinrichsen, G. A., Qualls, S. H., & Duffy, M. (2009). Pikes Peak Model for Training in Professional Geropsychology. *American Psychologist, 64,* 205–214.

Rodolfa, E., Bent, R., Eisman, E., Nelson, P. D., Rehm, L., & Ritchie, P. (2005). A cube model for competency development: Implications for psychology educators and regulators. *Professional Psychology: Research and Practice, 36,* 347–354.

The CoPGTP Task Force on Geropsychology Competency Assessment developed this tool. Task Force members are Michele J. Karel, Chair; Jeannette Berman, Jeremy Doughan, Erin E. Emery, Victor Molinari, Sarah Stoner, Yvette N. Tazeau, Susan K. Whitbourne, Janet Yang, and Richard Zweig.
Publications regarding tool development and evaluation:

Karel, M. J., Emery, E. E., & Molinari, V. (2010). Development of a tool to evaluate geropsychology knowledge and skill competencies. *International Psychogeriatrics, 22,* 886–896.

Karel, M. J., Holley, C. K., Whitbourne, S. K., Segal, D. L., Tazeau, Y. N., Emery, E. E., . . . Zweig, R. A. (2012). Preliminary validation of a tool to assess competencies for professional geropsychology practice. *Professional Psychology: Research and Practice, 43,* 110–117.

REFERENCES

American Bar Association Commission on Law and Aging and American Psychological Association. (2008). *Assessment of older adults with diminished capacity: A handbook for psychologists.* Washington, DC: Authors. Retrieved from http://www.apa.org/pi/aging

American Board of Geropsychology. (n.d.). *Geropsychology.* Retrieved from http://www.abpp.org/i4a/pages/index.cfm?pageid=3806

American Psychological Association. (2014). *Guidelines for psychological practice with older adults.* Retrieved from http://www.apa.org/practice/guidelines/older-adults.aspx

American Psychological Association, Division 20. (n.d.). *Division 20: Adult Development and Aging.* Retrieved from http://www.apadivisions.org/division-20

American Psychological Association, Office on Aging. (n.d.). *Office on Aging.* Retrieved from http://www.apa.org/pi/aging

Baltes, P. B., Lindenberger, U., & Staudinger, U. M. (1998). Life span theory in developmental psychology. In W. Damon (Series Ed.) & R. M. Lerner (Vol. Ed.), *Handbook of child psychology: Vol. 1. Theoretical models of human development* (5th ed., pp. 1029–1143). New York, NY: Wiley.

Council for Professional Training in Geropsychology. (n.d.). *The Council of Professional Geropsychology Training Programs (CoPGTP)*. Retrieved from http://www.copgtp.org/

Engel, G. L. (1977). The need for a new medical model: The challenge for biomedicine. *Science, 196*, 129–136. doi:10.1126/science.847460

France, C. R., Mastes, K. S., Belar, C. D., Kerns, R. D., Klonoff, E. A., Larkin, K. T., . . . Thorn, B. E. (2008). Application of the competency model to clinical health psychology. *Professional Psychology: Research and Practice, 39*, 573–580. doi:10.1037/0735-7028.39.6.573

Frankel, R. M., Quill, T. E., & McDaniel, S. H. (2003). *The biopsychosocial approach: past, present, and future*. Rochester, NY: University of Rochester Press.

Hannay, H. J., Bieliauskas, L., Crosson, B. A., Hammeke, T. A., & Hamsher, K. deS. & Koffler, S. (1998). Proceedings of the Houston conference on specialty education and training in clinical neuropsychology. *Archives of Clinical Neuropsychology, 13*, 157–250.

Jackson, Y., Wu, Y. P., Aylward, B. S., & Roberts, M. C. (2012). Application of the competency cube model to clinical child psychology. *Professional Psychology: Research and Practice, 43*, 432–441. doi:10.1037/a00300007

Karel, M. J., Emery, E. E., & Molinari, V. (2010). Development of a tool to evaluate geropsychology knowledge and skill competencies. *International Psychogeriatrics, 22*, 886–896. doi:10.1017/S1041610209991736

Karel, M. J., Holley, C. K., Whitbourne, S. K., Segal, D. L., Tazeau, Y. N., Emery, E. E., . . . Zweig, R. A. (2012). Preliminary validation of a tool to assess competencies for professional geropsychology practice. *Professional Psychology: Research and Practice, 43*, 110–117. doi:10.1037/a0025788

Karel, M. J., Knight, B. G., Duffy, M., Hinrichsen, G. A., & Zeiss, A. M. (2010). Attitude, knowledge, and skill competencies for practice in professional geropsychology: Implications for training and building a geropsychology workforce. *Training and Education in Professional Psychology, 4*, 75–84. doi:10.1037/a0018372.

Karlin, B. E., & Humphries, K. (2007). Improving Medicare coverage of psychological services for older Americans. *American Psychologist, 62*, 637–649. doi:10.1037/0003-066X.62.7.637

Kaslow, N. J. (2004). Competencies in professional psychology. *American Psychologist, 59*, 774–781. doi:10.1037/0003-066X.59.8.774

Knight, B. G. (2004). *Psychotherapy with older adults*. Thousand Oaks, CA: Sage.

Knight, B. G., Karel, M. J., Hinrichsen, G. A., Qualls, S. H., & Duffy, M. (2009). Pikes Peak model for training in professional geropsychology. *American Psychologist, 64*, 205–214. doi:10.1037/a0015059

Knight, G. B., Teri, L., Wohlford, P., & Santos, J. (Eds.). (1995). *Mental health services for older adults: Implications for training and practice in geropsychology*. Washington, DC: American Psychological Association. doi:10.1037/10184-000

Molinari, V. (Ed.). (2011). *Specialty competencies in geropsychology*. New York, NY: Oxford University Press.

Molinari, V. (2012). Application of the competency model to geropsychology. *Professional Psychology: Research and Practice, 43*, 403–409. doi:10.1037/a0026548

Psychologists in Long-Term Care, Inc. (n.d.). *PLTC-Psychologists in Long-Term Care, Inc*. Retrieved from http://www.pltcweb.org/index.php

Rey-Casserly, C., Roper, B. L., & Bauer, R. M. (2012). Application of a competency model to clinical neuropsychology. *Professional Psychology: Research and Practice, 43*, 422–431. doi:10.1037/a0028721.

Rodolfa, E. R., Bent, R. J., Eisman, E., Nelson, P. D., Rehm, L., & Ritchie, P. (2005). A cube model for competency development: Implications for psychology educators and regulators. *Professional Psychology: Research and Practice, 36*, 347–354. doi:10.1037/0735-7028.36.4.347

Santos, J. F., & VandenBos, G. R. (Eds.). (1982). *Psychology and the older adult: Challenges for training in the 1980s*. Washington, DC: American Psychological Association. doi:10.1037/10557-000

Scogin, F., & Shah, A. (Eds.). (2012). *Making evidence-based psychological treatments work with older adults*. Washington, DC: American Psychological Association. doi:10.1037/13753-000

Segal, D. L., Qualls, S. H., & Smyer, M. A. (2011). *Aging and mental health*. Oxford, England: Wiley-Blackwell.

Society of Clinical Geropsychology. (n.d.). *Welcome: Society of Clinical Geropsychology*. Retrieved from http://www.geropsychology.org/

Varela, J. G., & Conroy, M. A. (2012). Professional competencies in forensic psychology. *Professional Psychology: Research and Practice, 43*, 410–421. doi:10.1037/a0026776

2

COGNITIVE BEHAVIOR THERAPY AND BEHAVIORAL ACTIVATION FOR LATE-LIFE DEPRESSION

ELIZABETH A. DiNAPOLI, MICHAEL LaROCCA,
AND FORREST SCOGIN

In this chapter, we provide an overview of the evidence-based treatments of cognitive behavior therapy (CBT) and behavioral activation (BA) therapy for older adults with depression. We discuss the theoretical background, efficacy, and application of CBT and BA for late-life depression, and we provide a case example to illustrate these treatment techniques as they may apply to an actual client. We conclude with considerations for culture, disability, and cognitive impairment.

CASE EXAMPLE

R. G. is a 70-year-old European American, married man who presented to his primary care physician with the chief compliant of difficulties initiating and maintaining sleep. He often does not get to sleep until 12:00 a.m. and then wakes up at 4:00 a.m. and is unable to fall back asleep. His physician

http://dx.doi.org/10.1037/14524-003
Treatment of Late-Life Depression, Anxiety, Trauma, and Substance Abuse, P. A. Areán (Editor)

became concerned that R. G. may be experiencing secondary insomnia, which is characterized by sleep disturbances resulting from a medical disorder. R. G. is being treated for multiple medical comorbidities, such as arthritis, diabetes, and high blood pressure, that could disrupt his sleep. Furthermore, R. G. had prostate cancer a few years ago and was successfully treated. These health problems caused him to have some difficulty with completing day-to-day tasks, such as household chores. In addition, R. G. has recently experienced declines in his memory. On the St. Louis University Mental Status Examination (SLUMS; Tariq, Tumosa, Chibnall, Perry, & Morley, 2006), R. G.'s total score was 23 out of 30, below the normal range and suggesting mild cognitive decline.

Because he gets limited sleep, R. G. also reported that he often feels like he has no energy and has diminished interest in activities. Furthermore, when he gets up in the middle of the night, his frustration leads him to binge eat, which in turn increases his low self-esteem ("I'm tired of being fat, I look awful"). Because mental disorders commonly co-occur with symptoms of insomnia, the physician administered brief screeners for depression and anxiety. R. G. endorsed long-standing feelings of depression and anxiety. For example, he stated that he is unhappy, worthless, irritable/ tense, and generally pessimistic in his outlook on life. When asked to rate his mood on a 9-point scale (1 = *very depressed*; 9 = *very happy*), R. G. rated his mood a 2. However, he indicated he did not have suicidal or homicidal thoughts.

R. G. reported a family history of major depressive disorder (e.g., maternal uncle, male cousin, great grandmother). As a child, he was overweight and was often bullied and teased by his classmates because of his physical appearance. He stated that his low self-esteem and depression began in his childhood around age 12. During high school, R. G.'s confidence and mood improved when he developed close friends on the football team. However, when he entered college, he struggled with his grades ("I'm dumb") and peer relations, which exacerbated his depression. Even though R. G. struggled with depression, he successfully graduated from college and immediately afterward began working as an accountant. He described his job as extremely stressful, but he commented that he felt he was always being criticized by authority figures. R. G. has since retired, but he mentioned that he is still haunted by flashbacks about his job experience. In fact, he has persistent thoughts of being a failure in the workforce.

Currently, R. G. attributes his depression to being in an unhappy marriage, taking care of his ailing mother, and being restricted in the availability of pleasant activities. At the beginning of his marriage, R. G.'s wife cheated on him, and he continues to have doubts about her faithfulness. Recently, R. G.'s mother had a series of ministrokes, which has left her noncommunicative and in frail health. He visits his mother every other day in the nursing home, but he feels guilty because he thinks he should be doing more to help her. Due to his mother's poor health, R. G. cancelled the vacation he had planned for years and will not travel far from his home. Finally, R. G. lives in a rural area and often complains he is bored because of the lack of activities or entertainment. Since he retired, he finds that he spends the majority of his time watching TV and playing games on his computer. He has little meaningful engagement with other adults. In fact, R. G. dislikes socializing with more than two to three people in a group because it makes him nervous and he prefers to be by himself. R. G. was unable to identify any friends with whom he spends quality time.

THEORETICAL BACKGROUND OF COGNITIVE BEHAVIOR THERAPY

The fundamental premise of CBT is that how a person thinks, feels, and behaves determines how that person makes sense of their experiences (A. T. Beck, Rush, Shaw, & Emery, 1979). This premise is rooted in the writings of Greek philosophers such as Epictetus, who posited that people are not disturbed by things but by the views they take of them. Individuals have core beliefs that are a product of temperament and personal history. During times of stress, maladaptive core beliefs may generate negative automatic thoughts, which in turn yield emotions, sensations, and behaviors that compose the symptoms of mental distress (J. S. Beck, 1995). CBT encourages the client to engage in a process of discovery in which thoughts are identified as ideas or hypotheses to be tested rather than as beliefs that are fixed. This is done through cognitive and behavioral techniques such as thought identifying and monitoring; problem-solving techniques; activity scheduling; and examining and challenging core beliefs about the self, world, and future (Laidlaw, 2001).

Although derived primarily through the work of A. T. Beck (1967/1972; A. T. Beck et al., 1979), CBT has been adapted for use with older adults through protocols developed by Thompson, Dick-Siskin, Coon, Powers, and Gallagher-Thompson (2009). For older adults, CBT is an active, directive, time-limited, and structured treatment with the primary aim of symptom reduction (Laidlaw, Thompson, Dick-Siskin, & Gallagher-Thompson, 2003). The main goal of CBT is to improve the skills of older adults in examining and modifying maladaptive thoughts and beliefs. It is particularly suited to late-life depression because of its focus on symptoms such as inertia, hopelessness, and pessimism, especially in regard to health matters (Morris & Morris, 1991; Steuer & Hammen, 1983).

EFFICACY OF COGNITIVE BEHAVIOR
THERAPY FOR OLDER ADULTS

Several meta-analyses support the efficacy of CBT for older adults. In a meta-analysis of 122 psychotherapeutic intervention studies that included CBT, psychoanalysis, reminiscence, relaxation, and cognitive ability training among others, Pinquart and Sorensen (2001) found that CBT had above-average effects on depression and other self-ratings of subjective well-being among older adults. They also explored the factors affecting outcome, finding significant effects for longer treatment duration (i.e., more than nine sessions) and specialized therapist training in working with older adults. Moreover, in a meta-analysis of 57 controlled intervention studies, Pinquart, Duberstein, and Lyness (2007) found that CBT had large effect sizes for improvement in both self- and clinician-rated depression in older adults. Other meta-analyses of CBT for older adults (e.g., Cuijpers, van Straten, & Smit, 2006; Scogin & McElreath, 1994) indicate effect sizes ranging from 0.70 to 0.85, which are comparable to those of younger individuals in meta-analyses of cognitive behavioral approaches ($d = 0.72$; Michael & Crowley, 2002).

Randomized controlled trials have demonstrated the efficacy of CBT for late-life depression. Shah, Scogin, and Floyd (2012) found eight studies providing support for CBT as a beneficial and evidence-based treatment for depression in older adults (Campbell, 1992; Floyd, Scogin, McKendree-Smith, Floyd, & Rokke, 2004; Fry, 1984; Gallagher & Thompson, 1982; Gallagher-Thompson & Steffen, 1994; Laidlaw et al., 2008; Rokke, Tomhave, & Jocic, 1999; Thompson, Gallagher, & Breckenridge, 1987). These studies found CBT to be either superior to a control condition or not significantly different from another evidence-based treatment (behavioral therapy or brief psychodynamic therapy). In the study by Laidlaw et al., (2008), CBT was found to be nondifferentially efficacious as treatment as usual (TAU); both produced significant reductions in depressive symptoms immediately after treatment and 6 months posttreatment. However, an evaluation of outcome in terms of numbers of participants meeting research diagnostic criteria for depression yielded significant differences favoring the CBT condition at the end of treatment and at 4-month follow-up. In a study of older adults with depression who were in primary care, Serfaty et al., (2009) found that older adults receiving CBT had significantly lower Beck Depression Inventory-II scores than the TAU group. Moreover, in a sample of low-income older adults, Areán et al., (2005) found that clinical case management (CCM) and the combination of CCM with cognitive behavior group therapy (CBGT) led to greater improvements in depressive symptoms than CBGT alone. CBT also shows promise for older adults in rural areas. Scogin, Moss, Harris, and Presnell (2014) found home-delivered CBT to be superior to a minimal support control in reducing depressive symptoms among vulnerable, rural, predominately African American older adults.

CBT has also been shown to be as effective as or more effective than antidepressant medication in treating depression for older adults. In a meta-analysis of treatments for late-life depression, Pinquart, Duberstein, and Lyness (2006) found that CBT had a greater effect on clinician-rated depression than did selective serotonin reuptake inhibitors or other forms of psychotherapy. Another study compared the effects of CBT with those of desipramine in treating older adult outpatients with mild to moderate depression (Thompson, Coon, Gallagher-Thompson, Sommer, & Koin, 2001), finding that CBT-alone and combined groups had similar improvement. Specifically, the combined group showed greater improvement than the desipramine-alone group and the CBT-alone group also showed improvement. Older adults have also shown a preference for psychotherapy over medication. In a survey by Gum et al., (2006), more older adult patients preferred counseling (57%) than medication (43%) for treatment of depression, with previous experience of treatment type as the strongest predictor of preference.

Older adults have also been found to benefit from self-administered CBT. Scogin, Jamison, and Gochneaur (1989) compared the efficacy of cognitive and behavioral bibliotherapy for older adults with mild to moderate depression. Participants in the cognitive bibliotherapy condition read *Feeling Good* by Burns (1980) and learned such skills as understanding moods, changing feelings of guilt, and overcoming perfectionism, and those in the behavioral bibliotherapy group learned skills such as relaxation and activity planning. Scogin et al., (1989) found that both treatment groups were superior to the control condition, although the cognitive and behavioral groups were not differentially efficacious. Gains in treatment were maintained at 6-month follow-up. Other studies (e.g., Floyd, Scogin, McKendree-Smith, Floyd, & Rokke, 2004; Landreville & Bissonnette, 1997; Scogin, Hamblin, & Beutler, 1987) have provided further support for cognitive bibliotherapy as an evidence-based treatment for depression in older adults. These studies, like that of Scogin et al. (1989), used the book *Feeling Good* and allowed participants to work through the book at their own pace over approximately a 4-week period.

APPLICATION OF COGNITIVE BEHAVIOR THERAPY TO AGING-SPECIFIC ISSUES

According to Unützer, Katon, Sullivan, and Miranda (1999), chronic medical illness is the most important factor distinguishing older adults from those age 65 years or younger. Another critical factor is cognition. However, older adults are the least homogenous of all age groups, and they often have more dissimilarities than similarities (Dick & Gallagher-Thompson, 1995). There are at least two generations contained within this age grouping (Zeiss & Steffen, 1996b), and chronological age is an unreliable marker of whether age-specific therapeutic adaptations are necessary (Zeiss & Steffen, 1996a). As a result, therapists should attend to the functional status of the individual, rather than chronological age, when determining whether major adaptations are necessary. For older adults who do require adaptations, CBT is often appropriate because it may be modified in terms of pacing for cognitive slowing and changes in sensory perception (e.g., vision, hearing), without changing the substantive nature of the treatment (Laidlaw, 2001). CBT takes into account age-related changes in the understanding of problems (Thompson, 1996), and it can be modified to fit older adults' concerns such as grief, cognitive and physical limitations, and age-related depressive symptoms (Laidlaw, 2001). CBT may also help individuals to challenge negative attitudes toward aging by examining evidence for and against their beliefs while formulating alternative explanations for their thoughts (Laidlaw, 2010).

In an effort to maximize the potential for outcome in CBT for older adults, Laidlaw, Thompson, and Gallagher-Thompson (2001) developed a conceptual framework that added elements such as role transitions and investments, the sociocultural context, health status, cohort beliefs, and intergenerational relationships. This framework draws on gerontological theory to contextualize a person's problems within CBT while maintaining emphasis on interventions to optimize symptom reduction. Knight and Lee (2008) proposed a similar model of psychotherapy for older adults: the contextual adult life span theory for adapting psychotherapy (CALTAP) model. This model provides guidance of the specific nature of the context for older adults receiving psychotherapy, such as CBT, including specific social environments and the more macrolevel influences of culture and cohort (Knight & Poon, 2008).

CBT may also be well suited to the prevention of suicide in older adults. This is critical, given that male older adults in the United States have a higher rate of suicide than any other age group (Centers for Disease Control and Prevention, 2008). Bhar and Brown (2012) proposed a 12-session CBT protocol for reducing depression, suicidal ideation, and other risk factors of late-life suicide. Treatment includes assessing suicide risk, grasping the problem through a cognitive behavior framework, developing a safety plan, increasing hope and reasons for living, improving social resources, improving problem-solving skills, improving adherence to medical regimen, and preventing relapse.

Therapists face several challenges in conducting CBT with older adults. The experience of loss is a normal part of aging (Boerner & Jopp, 2007), and treatment of late-life depression may be challenging because of such losses as a death in the family or a loss of functioning due to declining health. Another challenge in treating late-life depression is that changes in appetite, poor sleep, and anhedonia may be in part caused by age-related physical and biological changes rather than depression (Laidlaw, 2010). Finally, older adults may avoid treatment because of negative stereotypes associated with aging (e.g., their problems arise from unchangeable personal attributes associated with aging).

THEORETICAL BACKGROUND OF BEHAVIORAL ACTIVATION

Depression often leads to a downward spiral in which feeling down causes a decrease in enjoyable activities, which in turn lowers mood further and continues to reduce activity level. This vicious tailspin pattern occurs with many older adults with depression. One way to reverse it is to engage in activities that bring a sense of pleasure or accomplishment. Referred to as behavioral activation (BA), this method targets changes in behavior as a way to improve thoughts, mood, and overall quality of life.

BA may be seen as an offshoot of the behavioral component of CBT. It is rooted in the behavioral theory of depression, which posits that depression is the result of not having sufficient positively reinforced experiences in the environment (Ferster, 1973; Lewinsohn, 1974; MacPhillamy & Lewinsohn, 1972). In keeping with this notion, BA has the goal of keeping patients active and engaged in life activities, rather than leading withdrawn, avoidant lifestyles (Snarski et al., 2011). It encourages individuals to explore how meaningful, reinforcing activities influence their mood (Martell, Addis, & Jacobson, 2001). The primary aim of BA for depression is for the individual to monitor mood and daily activities and to see their connection. Individuals then learn to develop a plan to increase the number of pleasant activities they engage in and to increase their positive interactions with their environment (Lazzari, Egan, & Rees, 2011). Attention is also given to improving the quality of their interactions with others to improve mood and feelings of self-control (Cuijpers, van Straten, & Warmerdam, 2007).

Hopko and colleagues (e.g., Lejuez, Hopko, & Hopko, 2001) have modified BA treatment into a shorter, simpler approach that adjusts the original BA protocol to adhere more closely to behavioral techniques. This brief BA treatment for depression (BATD) does not emphasize the cognitive-based techniques that may be used in BA. Rather, patients and practitioners collaborate to identify individualized target behaviors, goals, and rewards that reinforce nondepressive or healthy behavior. Specifically, patients are asked to rate their life goals and values on a chart, after which they create an activity hierarchy, with 15 activities that are rated from *easiest* to *most difficult* (Hopko, Bell, Armento, Hunt, & Lejuez, 2005). The patient progresses in the therapy from the easy to the more challenging tasks, and the final goal is to increase the frequency and duration of the activities.

Riebe, Fan, Unützer, and Vannoy (2012) examined the participant records from the Improving Mood-Promoting Access to Collaborative Treatment trial (Unützer et al., 2002) to investigate the specific types of activities in activity scheduling for optimal treatment outcomes. Results indicated a positive association between pleasant activity engagement and depression improvement at 12 months. More specifically, older adults tended to focus on scheduling the following activities: physical activity/exercise (32%); medication management (22%); and active, nonphysical activities (19%). In addition, activities that involved interacting with family or engaging in interpersonal exchange ("socialize") had the most improved depression outcomes.

EFFICACY OF BEHAVIORAL ACTIVATION FOR OLDER ADULTS

In an early study of the utility of BA, Jacobson et al. (1996) found that full CBT did not add benefits over receiving BA alone. They speculated that the exposure to naturally reinforcing contingencies in BA produces changes in thinking more effectively than do purely cognitive interventions. More recently, in a randomized treatment trial, Dimidjian et al. (2006) found BA to be comparable to antidepressant medication and more effective than CBT among adults with more severe depression. Neither of these studies included older adult participants.

Behavioral treatments often emphasize patient pleasant events, and such treatments have demonstrated efficacy in settings such as nursing homes, assisted living facilities, and geriatric psychiatry facilities. For instance, the Behavioral Activities Intervention (BE-ACTIV) is a behavioral intervention for depression in nursing homes that emphasizes activation and engagement in pleasant events (Meeks, Looney, Van Haitsma, & Teri, 2008). Results of two trial phases of this intervention suggest that BE-ACTIV reduces institutional barriers to participation in pleasant activities, increases residents' control over activity participation, increases overall activity participation, and reduces depressive symptoms. Pleasant events-focused BA has also benefited patients with dementia. In a controlled clinical trial of behavioral treatment for depression in patients with dementia, Teri, Logsdon, Uomoto, and McCurry (1997) found that emphasizing patient pleasant events showed significant improvement in depressive symptoms compared to control and typical care conditions, with gains maintained at follow up. Among assisted living patients, Cernin and Lichtenberg (2009) found that a pleasant events intervention delivered by assisted living staff to senior residents over a 3-month period resulted in reduced depressive symptoms and increased subjective global mood.

In a case study of a nursing home resident with recurrent major depression, Meeks, Teri, Van Haitsma, and Looney (2006) evaluated the efficacy of a 10-session BA program involving negotiating a weekly plan to systematically increase pleasant activities. They found that the treatment markedly improved positive affect, increased activity level at posttreatment, and significantly reduced depressive symptoms at posttreatment and at 12-week follow-up. Results were similar in a study by Yon and Scogin (2008), which found that in-home BA therapy significantly reduced depression in older adults. Treatment included components such as increasing pleasant events and decreasing dysfunctional attitudes through targeting behavior, and 71% of participants no longer met criteria for a depressive disorder at posttreatment. More recently, Snarski et al. (2011) found that BA significantly reduced depressive symptoms in older adult psychiatric inpatients.

APPLICATION OF BEHAVIORAL ACTIVATION TO AGING-SPECIFIC ISSUES

BA appears to be well suited to older adults. Due to the failing health and the increasing physical limitations that accompany aging, activities enjoyed as a younger adult may be abandoned. Benyamini and Lomranz (2004) argued that this activity restriction is related to depressive symptoms. BA may aid in reducing these symptoms by encouraging older adults to become more active (Yon & Scogin, 2008). According to Blazer (2002), BA encourages clients to recognize feelings of accomplishment through completing daily activities, which may in turn decrease symptoms of depression by increasing self-efficacy. Moreover, the relatively straightforward nature of BA may make it more easily understood by older adults with low education levels or with mild cognitive impairment (Porter, Spates, & Smitham, 2004). Hertzog and Hultsch (2000) noted that older adults have more difficulty reframing and controlling their thoughts than do younger adults, which further suggests that BA may be a more effective treatment for older adults than more cognitively driven techniques.

Various instruments may be used to assess the extent to which older adults make use of pleasant events, and these instruments may in turn inspire greater activity. For example, the California Older Person's Pleasant Events Schedule (COPPES; Rider, Gallagher-Thompson, & Thompson, 2004) asks the individual to rate the subjective pleasantness of 66 events and the degree to which he or she participates in them. Completion of this questionnaire provides the clinician with a more complete analysis of the functioning of an older adult with depression, and steps may then be taken to help the individual do more of the activities he or she finds enjoyable. Alternatively, the 20-item Pleasant Events Scale (PES; Teri & Lewinsohn, 1982) is a shorter questionnaire asking the individual to rate pleasant events (e.g., "Seeing beautiful scenery," "Talking about my children or grandchildren"). Like the COPPES, the PES may be used to evaluate pleasant events as mediators of change in depression (Yon & Scogin, 2008).

APPLICATION TO CASE EXAMPLE

CBT should be introduced with a thorough explanation of the four central components (thoughts, feelings, behaviors, and physiology) of this approach. To illustrate how these four components are intertwined, the therapist asked R. G. to describe his most recent stressful event, which was visiting his ailing mother in the nursing home. R. G. described the event of going to the nursing home as dreadful (feeling), which was associated with thoughts such as "I'm a bad son," "She is going to die soon," and "I don't do enough to help my mother." These thoughts and feelings decreased R. G.'s motivation to visit his mother (behavior) and led him to feel tension throughout his body. Because R. G. felt tension in his body, he decided to lie in bed all afternoon (behavior). Therefore, his thinking was related to the way he felt and how he reacted to the event. By working through this example, R. G. was able to understand how these four components interact with one another to produce depression (see Figure 2.1). Because psychotherapy cannot directly change

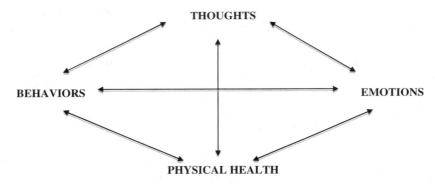

Figure 2.1. The four components of the cognitive behavior therapy model. From *Treating Late-Life Depression: A Cognitive-Behavioral Therapy Approach, Workbook* (p. 5), by L. W. Thompson, L. Dick-Siskin, D. W. Coon, D. V. Powers, and D. Gallagher-Thompson, 2009, New York, NY: Oxford University Press. Copyright 2009 by Oxford University Press. Reprinted with permission.

feelings and physiology (body), the therapist focuses on changing behaviors by building in more reinforcing activities (BA) and changing unhelpful thoughts by challenging their adaptiveness (CBT).

Application of Behavioral Activation to Case Example

An early task of BA is to get an accurate assessment of the client's current daily schedule of activities. For example, R. G. was asked to keep a detailed record (every 2 hours) of all the activities he engaged in for 2 to 3 days. By doing this, R. G. was able to realize that he was doing less than he thought, which inspired him to develop some ideas about activities he would like to add to his schedule. R. G. was also given a list of activities that older adults tend to enjoy and was asked to identify activities that he finds pleasurable. He identified six rewarding and pleasurable activities in which he would like to more frequently engage: (a) looking at beautiful scenery (e.g., sunset and clouds), (b) listening to audiobooks, (c) volunteering at the hospital, (d) taking digital photography, (e) working out at the gym (e.g., tai chi, running, weight lifting), and (f) going to church. R. G. chose the frequency with which he would like to engage in each activity and then made plans on how he would incorporate these activities into his weekly schedule.

An important part of BA is to integrate monitoring mood with identifying pleasant events. Because R. G. often described his mood as either "depressed" or "happy," he was asked to rate his mood on a 9-point Likert scale as a way for him to notice the "in-between." Recognizing the in-between helped him pay attention to his mood ratings and the activities that made his mood better or worse. Finally, R. G. was asked to rate his mood and write a description of why he thought he felt this way. This allowed him to recognize the activities that contributed more to his mood ratings, as well as confirmed that greater engagement in pleasant events was related to a better mood rating.

Application of Cognitive Behavior Therapy to Case Example

An integral assumption of CBT is that unhelpful thoughts create negative emotions. Yet, this process happens so quickly that the thoughts that occur between a stressful event and difficult emotions go unrecognized. These thoughts are called automatic thoughts, because they appear so fast and go unnoticed unless a conscious effort is made to notice them. Therefore, CBT aims to slow down the thought processes to identify the cognitive processes associated with negative emotional reactions.

R. G. started challenging his unhelpful thoughts by filling out a three-column Unhelpful Thought Diary (UTD), which required him to identify a stressful event, the automatic thoughts that accompanied it, and his emotional reaction to the distressing event. He was then able to identify the negative thoughts ("I will never be able to sleep like a normal person again! I'm wide awake and I have to wake up in four hours") that occur when he has difficulty falling asleep at night, which in turn made him feel helpless and angry. Therefore, R. G. learned how to monitor the thoughts that immediately follow his difficulty initiating sleep.

As R. G. became more aware of his unhelpful thoughts, it was important to begin introducing techniques for challenging their veracity. He learned multiple techniques for challenging his unhelpful thoughts, but he found examining the consequences of keeping his negative thoughts, doing things to obtain extra information, and considering the in-betweens of results the most useful. For example, R. G. discussed the consequences of holding onto the thought "I will never be able to sleep like a normal person again" while trying to fall asleep. He recognized that this worrying only made him more tense and frustrated, and this made it harder for him to fall asleep. These techniques allowed R. G. to determine whether his thoughts were factual or just exaggerations based on incomplete information.

Once R. G. learned techniques to identify his unhelpful thoughts, the three-column UTD needed to be expanded to include two additional columns to list more realistic thoughts and ratings of new emotions (five-column UTD). R. G. was able to replace his original unhelpful thought with "There is no point in lying here worrying about how much sleep I'll get"; "I can't force myself to sleep anyway"; and "Worrying about it will only make me more tense and wide awake, so it will be even harder to fall back asleep." In addition, R. G. acknowledged that even on the most horrible night of sleep, he was still able to function adequately the next day. Therefore, instead of feeling helpless and angry, his emotions changed to hopeful and relaxed. In sum, CBT taught R. G. to turn around his thoughts to gain new perspectives and more adaptive beliefs that lead to more helpful emotions.

CONSIDERATIONS FOR CULTURE, DISABILITY, AND COGNITIVE IMPAIRMENT

The population of the United States is growing older and more ethnically diverse (Crowther, Shurgot, Perkins, & Rodriguez, 2006). In 2010, 20% of older adults in the United States were from ethnic minority cultures, representing over a 300% increase in the older ethnic minority population since the late 1990s (American Association of Retired Persons, 2011; Haley, Han, & Henderson, 1998). Moreover, great diversity exists within ethnic groups in terms of culture, language, immigration and acculturation histories, and life experiences based on cohorts (Lau & Kinoshita, 2006).

As part of the CALTAP model, Knight and Poon (2008) noted that older adults' approach to psychotherapy may be influenced by their cultural values and beliefs. These include illness interpretation, attitude toward help seeking, and presentation in therapy. According to Knight and Poon, non-Western ethnic minority older adults may interpret illness on the basis of underlying assumptions that differ from those of Westerners. They provided the example of minorities from Southeast Asia who view individuals as part of a larger social context rather than a mind–body duality. This example applies to many other cultures in Asia and elsewhere that take a collectivistic view of society, rather than the individualistic view that is typical of Western countries. Knight and Poon noted that ethnic minority older adults might be less inclined to seek help because of fears of shame and stigma. They are also more likely to present in somatic rather than psychological terms, as bodily complaints are perceived as carrying less stigma than problems in mental health. Therapists must be sensitive to these cultural differences and be prepared to adjust treatment accordingly.

Although studies of the cultural implications of BA for older adults are lacking, a growing body of research exists on CBT for ethnic minorities. Horrell (2008) identified six studies that reported findings of CBT as a treatment for ethnic minority adults with depression. These minority groups included low-income ethnic minorities (Organista, Muñoz, & González, 1994), low-income ethnic minority women (Miranda et al., 2003), Hispanic women (Gelman, López, & Foster, 2006; Lara, Navarro, Rubí, & Mondragón, 2003), African Americans (Markowitz, Spielman, Sullivan, & Fishman, 2000), and older Chinese Americans (Dai et al., 1999). Results of these studies are promising, particularly for Hispanic/Latina and African American women, whereas less information exists regarding the use of CBT with Hispanic/Latino men. Moreover, results were inconclusive for Chinese Americans and African American men. Only the study by Dai et al. (1999) focused on older adults. Whether the results of the other studies generalize to older ethnic minority adults is unclear, particularly those who do not speak English and may be less assimilated to the new culture than their younger counterparts.

According to Comas-Díaz (2011), cultural adaptation in psychotherapy has alternated between adapting psychotherapy systems to marginalized populations (culturally adapted psychotherapy) and developing new systems of psychotherapy to better fit marginalized client populations (ethnic and indigenous psychotherapies). Researchers have suggested cultural modifications to treatment, including multicultural training for therapists (Hays, 1995), ethnic matching of the therapist and client (S. Sue, Fujino, Hu, Takeuchi, & Zane, 1991), addressing cultural differences at the outset of therapy, conducting therapy in an important cultural setting, and conducting therapy in the client's native language (D. W. Sue & Sue, 2003). However, only ethnic matching and multicultural training have been studied empirically, with mixed results. For example, Presnell, Harris, and Scogin (2012) found no evidence of ethnic match on process or outcome variables in a study of African American and European American older adults and psychotherapists. Nevertheless, many researchers suggest it is important to train psychologists to be culturally competent to improve recruitment and retention of ethnic minorities in research and improve therapy outcomes (Hays, 1995; S. Sue, 1998; Toporek & Pope-Davis, 2005). A meta-analysis of multicultural training suggested that such training significantly increases participants' multicultural competence (Smith, Constantine, Dunn, Dinehart, & Montoya, 2006). Therapist cultural competence is even more important with older adult clients, who may have more traditional views of psychotherapy (e.g., stigma associated with mental health treatment), than their younger counterparts.

Older adults with depression and with cognitive impairment may benefit from BA. For example, increasing pleasant activities among dementia patients has been shown to reduce depression (e.g., Teri et al., 1997; Teri & Uomoto, 1991). Moreover, both CBT and BA may be modified to fit the cognitive impairment, physical limitations, and lack of mobility that afflict many older adults. One such modification of CBT is that developed by Thompson, Gallagher-Thompson, and Dick (1995), which includes activity scheduling, changing unhelpful thoughts, relaxation, and assertiveness. The modification also includes providing in-session cue cards as memory aids, slowing down the pace of the intervention, and simplifying the homework assignments. In a CBT intervention of frail, rural older adults, Scogin et al. (2007) used Thompson et al.'s (1995) modifications with promising results, finding significant improvements in quality of life and reductions in psychological symptoms. A secondary analysis of these data also revealed significant reductions in depressive symptoms (Scogin et al., 2014).

In their CBT protocol for depression and suicide in older adults, Bhar and Brown (2012) used additional techniques to accommodate for disabilities. These included taking frequent breaks during sessions, writing key points and agenda items on a whiteboard, using brief versions of self-report questionnaires to accommodate limitations in attention span, providing frequent capsule summaries to remind the patient of the issue discussed and conclusion reached, and reviewing the past session at the start of each new therapy session. For patients with transportation difficulties, Bhar and Brown suggested that clinicians help organize transportation, arrange for some sessions to be conducted by phone and that they have sessions coincide with other nearby appointments if possible. Treatment may also be augmented through the use of case management services (Areán, Hegel, & Reynolds, 2001). These services include coordinating treatment with the patient's medical appointments and establishing linkages to social, community, and financial services.

CONCLUSION

The case of R. G. lends itself well to the workings of CBT and BA. He is a European American older adult who has depression, insomnia, anxiety, and poor self-esteem, and his problems are exacerbated by his strained marital relationship and his mother's poor health. CBT helped him to understand how his feelings of worthlessness and guilt may lead to his inability to fall asleep, which in turn leads to his binge eating followed by feelings of low self-esteem. CBT's attention to reframing unhelpful thoughts helped R. G. to stall and then reverse his cycle of negative thoughts and behaviors. CBT is also flexible in its approach and may be fitted to his needs as an older adult (e.g., making modifications for pace and cognitive slowing, as necessary). After 10 sessions, R. G. showed notable improvement in challenging his negative automatic thoughts dealing with insomnia along with guilt over his role as a son. By replacing these thoughts with more positive self-statements, R. G. slept more soundly and reported fewer depressive symptoms.

R. G.'s age and his restriction in pleasant activities also made him a good candidate for BA. By understanding the connection between pleasant activities and improved mood, R. G. gained increased incentive to plan simple, rewarding activities appropriate to his lifestyle and level of functioning. Toward the end of his course of treatment, these activities reduced his feelings of depression and increased his self-efficacy. His renewed self-esteem assisted in easing the tensions with his wife while assuaging his guilty feelings concerning his mother.

REFERENCES

American Association of Retired Persons. (2011). *A profile of older Americans: 2011.* Washington, DC: U.S. Department of Health and Human Services.

Areán, P. A., Gum, A., McCulloch, C. E., Bostrom, A., Gallagher-Thompson, D., & Thompson, L. (2005). Treatment of depression in low-income older adults. *Psychology and Aging, 20,* 601–609. doi:10.1037/0882-7974.20.4.601

Areán, P. A., Hegel, M., & Reynolds, C. (2001). Treating depression in older medical patients with psychotherapy. *Journal of Clinical Geropsychology, 7,* 93–104. doi:10.1023/A:1009581504993

Beck, A. T. (1972). *Depression: Causes and treatment.* Philadelphia: University of Pennsylvania Press. (Original work published 1967)

Beck, A. T., Rush, A. J., Shaw, B. F., & Emery, G. (1979). *Cognitive therapy of depression*. New York, NY: Guilford Press.

Beck, J. S. (1995). *Cognitive therapy: Basics and beyond*. New York, NY: Guilford Press.

Benyamini, Y., & Lomranz, J. (2004). The relationship of activity restriction and replacement with depressive symptoms among older adults. *Psychology and Aging, 19*, 362–366. doi:10.1037/0882-7974.19.2.362

Bhar, S. S., & Brown, G. K. (2012). Treatment of depression and suicide in older adults. *Cognitive and Behavioral Practice, 19*, 116–125. doi:10.1016/j.cbpra.2010.12.005

Blazer, D. G. (2002). Self-efficacy and depression in late life: A primary prevention proposal. *Aging & Mental Health, 6*, 315–324. doi:10.1080/1360786021000006938

Boerner, K., & Jopp, D. A. (2007). Improvement/maintenance and reorientation as central features of coping with major life change and loss: Contributions of three major life-span theories. *Human Development, 50*, 171–195. doi:10.1159/000103358

Burns, D. D. (1980). *Feeling good*. New York, NY: Avon Books.

Campbell, J. M. (1992). Treating depression in well older adults: Use of diaries in cognitive therapy. *Issues in Mental Health Nursing, 13*, 19–29. doi:10.3109/01612849209006882

Centers for Disease Control and Prevention. (2008). Web-Based Injury Statistics Query and Reporting System (WISQARS). Retrieved from http://webappa.cdc.gov/sasweb/ncipc/mortrate10_sy.html

Cernin, P., & Lichtenberg, P. (2009). Behavioral treatment for depressed mood: A pleasant events intervention for seniors residing in assisted living. *Clinical Gerontologist, 32*, 324–331. doi:10.1080/07317110902896547

Comas-Díaz, L. (2011). Multicultural approaches to psychotherapy. In J. C. Norcross, G. R. VandenBos, & D. K. Freedheim (Eds.), *History of psychotherapy: Continuity and change* (2nd ed., pp. 243–267). Washington, DC: American Psychological Association. doi:10.1037/12353-008

Crowther, M. R., Shurgot, G., Perkins, M., & Rodriguez, R. (2006). The social and cultural context of psychotherapy with older adults. In S. H. Qualls & B. G. Knight (Eds.), *Psychotherapy for depression in older adults* (pp. 179–199). Hoboken, NJ: Wiley.

Cuijpers, P., van Straten, A., & Smit, F. (2006). Psychological treatment of late life depression: A meta-analysis of randomized controlled trials. *International Journal of Geriatric Psychiatry, 21*, 1139–1149. doi:10.1002/gps.1620

Cuijpers, P., van Straten, A., & Warmerdam, L. (2007). Behavioral activation treatments of depression: A meta-analysis. *Clinical Psychology Review, 27*, 318–326. doi:10.1016/j.cpr.2006.11.001

Dai, Y., Zhang, S., Yamamoto, J., Ao, M., Belin, T. R., Cheung, F., & Hifumi, S. S. (1999). Cognitive behavioral therapy of minor depressive symptoms in elderly Chinese Americans: A pilot study. *Community Mental Health Journal, 35*, 537–542. doi:10.1023/A:1018763302198

Dick, L. P., & Gallagher-Thompson, D. (1995). Cognitive therapy with the core beliefs of a distressed lonely caregiver. *Journal of Cognitive Psychotherapy, 9,* 215–227.

Dimidjian, S., Hollon, S. D., Dobson, K. S., Schmaling, K. B., Kohlenberg, R. J., Addis, M. E., . . . Jacobson, N. S. (2006). Randomized trial of behavioral activation, cognitive therapy, and antidepressant medication in the acute treatment of adults with major depression. *Journal of Consulting and Clinical Psychology, 74,* 658–670. doi:10.1037/0022-006X.74.4.658

Ferster, C. B. (1973). A functional analysis of depression. *American Psychologist, 28,* 857–870. doi:10.1037/h0035605

Floyd, M., Scogin, F., McKendree-Smith, N. L., Floyd, D. L., & Rokke, P. D. (2004). Cognitive therapy for depression: A comparison of individual psychotherapy and bibliotherapy for depressed older adults. *Behavior Modification, 28,* 297–318. doi:10.1177/0145445503259284

Fry, P. S. (1984). Cognitive training and cognitive-behavioral variables in the treatment of depression in the elderly. *Clinical Gerontologist, 3,* 25–45. doi:10.1300/J018v03n01_04

Gallagher, D. E., & Thompson, L. W. (1982). Treatment of major depressive disorder in older adult outpatients with brief psychotherapies. *Psychotherapy: Theory, Research, & Practice, 19,* 482–490. doi:10.1037/h0088461

Gallagher-Thompson, D., & Steffen, A. M. (1994). Comparative effects of cognitive-behavioral and brief psychodynamic psychotherapies for depressed family caregivers. *Journal of Consulting and Clinical Psychology, 62,* 543–549. doi:10.1037/0022-006X.62.3.543

Gelman, C. R., López, M., & Foster, R. P. (2006). Evaluating the impact of a cognitive–behavioral intervention with depressed Latinas: A preliminary report. *Social Work in Mental Health, 4,* 1–16. doi:10.1300/J200v04n02_01

Gum, A. M., Areán, P. A., Hunkeler, E., Tang, L., Katon, W., Hitchcock, P., . . . Unützer, J. (2006). Depression treatment preferences in older primary care patients. *The Gerontologist, 46,* 14–22. doi:10.1093/geront/46.1.14

Haley, W. E., Han, B., & Henderson, J. (1998). Aging and ethnicity: Issues for clinical practice. *Journal of Clinical Psychology in Medical Settings, 5,* 393–409. doi:10.1023/A:1026266422665

Hays, P. A. (1995). Multicultural applications of cognitive–behavior therapy. *Professional Psychology: Research and Practice, 26,* 309–315. doi:10.1037/0735-7028.26.3.309

Hertzog, C., & Hultsch, D. F. (2000). Metacognition in adulthood and old age. In C. Fergus & T. A. Salthouse (Eds.), *Handbook of aging and cognition* (pp. 417–466). Mahwah, NJ: Erlbaum.

Hopko, D. R., Bell, J. L., Armento, M. E. A., Hunt, M. K., & Lejuez, C. W. (2005). Behavior therapy for depressed cancer patients in primary care. *Psychotherapy: Theory, Research, Practice, Training, 42,* 236–243. doi:10.1037/0033-3204.42.2.236

Horrell, S. (2008). Effectiveness of cognitive-behavioral therapy with adult ethnic minority clients: A review. *Professional Psychology: Research and Practice, 39,* 160–168. doi:10.1037/0735-7028.39.2.160

Jacobson, N. S., Dobson, K. S., Truax, P. A., Addis, M. E., Koerner, K., Gollan, J. K., . . . Prince, S. E. (1996). A component analysis of cognitive-behavioral treatment for depression. *Journal of Consulting and Clinical Psychology, 64,* 295–304. doi:10.1037/0022-006X.64.2.295

Knight, B. G., & Lee, L. O. (2008). Contextual adult life span theory for adapting psychotherapy. In K. Laidlaw & B. G. Knight (Eds.), *Handbook of emotional disorders in late life: Assessment and treatment* (pp. 59–88). Oxford, England: Oxford University Press.

Knight, B. G., & Poon, C. M. (2008). Contextual adult life span theory for adapting psychotherapy with older adults. *Journal of Rational-Emotive & Cognitive-Behavior Therapy, 26,* 232–249. doi:10.1007/s10942-008-0084-7

Laidlaw, K. (2001). An empirical review of cognitive therapy for late life depression: Does research evidence suggest adaptations are necessary for cognitive therapy with older adults? *Clinical Psychology & Psychotherapy, 8,* 1–14. doi:10.1002/cpp.276

Laidlaw, K. (2010). Are attitudes to ageing and wisdom enhancement legitimate targets for CBT for late life depression and anxiety? *Nordic Psychology, 62,* 27–42. doi:10.1027/1901-2276/a000009

Laidlaw, K., Davidson, K. M., Toner, H. L., Jackson, G., Clark, S., Law, J., . . . Connery, H. (2008). A randomised controlled trial of cognitive behaviour therapy versus treatment as usual in the treatment of mild to moderate late life depression. *International Journal of Geriatric Psychiatry, 23,* 843–850. doi:10.1002/gps.1993

Laidlaw, K., Thompson, L. W., Dick-Siskin, L., & Gallagher-Thompson, D. (2003). *Cognitive behaviour therapy with older people.* Chichester, England: Wiley. doi:10.1002/9780470713402

Laidlaw, K., Thompson, L. W., & Gallagher-Thompson, D. (2001). Comprehensive conceptualization of cognitive behaviour therapy for late life depression. *Behavioural and Cognitive Psychotherapy, 32,* 389–399. doi:10.1017/S1352465804001584

Landreville, P., & Bissonnette, L. (1997). Effects of cognitive bibliotherapy for depressed older adults with a disability. *Clinical Gerontologist, 17,* 35–55. doi:10.1300/J018v17n04_05

Lara, M. A., Navarro, C., Rubí, N. A., & Mondragón, L. (2003). Outcome results of two levels of intervention in low-income women with depressive symptoms. *American Journal of Orthopsychiatry, 73,* 35–43. doi:10.1037/0002-9432.73.1.35

Lau, A. W., & Kinoshita, L. M. (2006). Cognitive-behavioral therapy with culturally diverse older adults. In P. A. Hays & G. Y. Iwamasa (Eds.), *Culturally responsive cognitive-behavioral therapy: Assessment, practice, and supervision* (pp. 179–197). Washington, DC: American Psychological Association. doi:10.1037/11433-008

Lazzari, C., Egan, S. J., & Rees, C. S. (2011). Behavioral activation treatment for depression in older adults delivered via videoconferencing: A pilot study. *Cognitive and Behavioral Practice, 18,* 555–565. doi:10.1016/j.cbpra.2010.11.009

Lejuez, C. W., Hopko, D. R., & Hopko, S. D. (2001). A brief behavioral activation treatment for depression: Treatment manual. *Behavior Modification, 25,* 255–286. doi:10.1177/0145445501252005

Lewinsohn, P. (1974). A behavioral approach to depression. In R. Friedman & M. Katz (Eds.), *The psychology of depression: Contemporary theory and research* (pp. 157–176). New York, NY: Wiley.

MacPhillamy, D. J., & Lewinsohn, P. M. (1972). The measurement of reinforcing events. In: *Proceedings of the 80th Annual Convention of the American Psychological Association, 7,* 399–400.

Markowitz, J. C., Spielman, L. A., Sullivan, M., & Fishman, B. (2000). An exploratory study of ethnicity and psychotherapy outcome among HIV-positive patients with depressive symptoms. *The Journal of Psychotherapy Practice and Research, 9,* 226–231.

Martell, C. R., Addis, M. E., & Jacobson, N. S. (2001). *Depression in context: Strategies for guided action.* New York, NY: Norton.

Meeks, S., Looney, S. W., Van Haitsma, K. W., & Teri, L. (2008). BE-ACTIV: A staff-assisted behavioral intervention for depression in nursing homes. *The Gerontologist, 48,* 105–114. doi:10.1093/geront/48.1.105

Meeks, S., Teri, L., Van Haitsma, K., & Looney, S. (2006). Increasing pleasant events in the nursing home: Collaborative behavioral treatment for depression. *Clinical Case Studies, 5,* 287–304. doi:10.1177/1534650104267418

Michael, K. D., & Crowley, S. L. (2002). How effective are treatments for child and adolescent depression? A meta-analytic review. *Clinical Psychology Review, 22,* 247–269. doi:10.1016/S0272-7358(01)00089-7

Miranda, J., Chung, J. Y., Green, B. L., Krupnick, J., Siddique, J., Revicki, D. A., & Belin, T. (2003). Treating depression in predominately low-income young minority women: A randomized controlled trial. *JAMA, 290,* 57–65. doi:10.1001/jama.290.1.57

Morris, R. G., & Morris, L. W. (1991). Cognitive and behavioural approaches with the depressed elderly. *International Journal of Geriatric Psychiatry, 6,* 407–413. doi:10.1002/gps.930060612

Organista, K. C., Muñoz, R. F., & González, G. (1994). Cognitive behavioral therapy for depression in low-income and minority medical outpatients: Description of a program and exploratory analyses. *Cognitive Therapy and Research, 18,* 241–259. doi:10.1007/BF02357778

Pinquart, M., Duberstein, P. R., & Lyness, J. M. (2006). Treatments for later-life depressive conditions: A meta-analytic comparison of pharmacotherapy and psychotherapy. *The American Journal of Psychiatry, 163,* 1493–1501. doi:10.1176/appi.ajp.163.9.1493

Pinquart, M., Duberstein, P. R., & Lyness, J. M. (2007). Effects of psychotherapy and other behavioral interventions on clinically depressed older adults: A meta-analysis. *Aging & Mental Health, 11*, 645–657. doi:10.1080/13607860701529635

Pinquart, M., & Sorensen, S. (2001). How effective are psychotherapeutic and other psychosocial interventions with older adults? A meta-analysis. *Journal of Mental Health and Aging, 7*, 207–243.

Porter, J. F., Spates, C., & Smitham, S. (2004). Behavioral activation group therapy in public mental health settings: A pilot investigation. *Professional Psychology: Research and Practice, 35*, 297–301. doi:10.1037/0735-7028.35.3.297

Presnell, A., Harris, G., & Scogin, F. (2012). Therapist and client race/ethnicity match: An examination of treatment outcome and process with rural older adults in the deep south. *Psychotherapy Research, 22*, 458–463. doi:10.1080/105 03307.2012.673022

Rider, K. L., Gallagher-Thompson, D., & Thompson, L. W. (2004). *California Older Person's Pleasant Events Schedule: Manual.* Retrieved from http://oafc.stanford. edu/coppes_files/Manual2.pdf

Riebe, G., Fan, M.-Y., Unützer, J., & Vannoy, S. (2012). Activity scheduling as a core component of effective care management for late-life depression. *International Journal of Geriatric Psychiatry, 27*, 1298–1304. doi:10.1002/gps.3784

Rokke, P. D., Tomhave, J. A., & Jocic, Z. (1999). The role of client choice and target selection in self-management therapy for depression in older adults. *Psychology and Aging, 14*, 155–169. doi:10.1037/0882-7974.14.1.155

Scogin, F., Hamblin, D., & Beutler, L. (1987). Bibliotherapy for depressed older adults: A self-help alternative. *The Gerontologist, 27*, 383–387. doi:10.1093/geront/27.3.383

Scogin, F., Jamison, C., & Gochneaur, K. (1989). Comparative efficacy of cognitive and behavioral bibliotherapy for mildly and moderately depressed older adults. *Journal of Consulting and Clinical Psychology, 57*, 403–407. doi:10.1037/0022-006X.57.3.403

Scogin, F., & McElreath, L. (1994). Efficacy of psychosocial treatments for geriatric depression: A quantitative review. *Journal of Consulting and Clinical Psychology, 62*, 69–74. doi:10.1037/0022-006X.62.1.69

Scogin, F., Morthland, M., Kaufman, A., Burgio, L., Chaplin, W., & Kong, G. (2007). Improving quality of life in diverse rural older adults: A randomized trial of a psychological treatment. *Psychology and Aging, 22*, 657–665. doi:10.1037/0882-7974.22.4.657

Scogin, F. R., Moss, K., Harris, G. M., & Presnell, A. H. (2014). Treatment of depressive symptoms in diverse, rural, and vulnerable older adults. *International Journal of Geriatric Psychiatry, 29*, 310–316. doi:10.1002/gps.4009.

Serfaty, M. A., Haworth, D., Blanchard, M., Buszewicz, M., Murad, S., & King, M. (2009). Clinical effectiveness of individual cognitive behavioral therapy for depressed older people in primary care: A randomized controlled trial. *Archives of General Psychiatry, 66*, 1332–1340. doi:10.1001/archgenpsychiatry.2009.165

Shah, A., Scogin, F., & Floyd, M. (2012). Evidence-based psychological treatments for geriatric depression. In F. Scogin & A. Shah (Eds.), *Making evidence-based psychological treatments work with older adults* (pp. 87–130). Washington, DC: American Psychological Association. doi:10.1037/13753-004

Smith, T. B., Constantine, M. G., Dunn, T. W., Dinehart, J. M., & Montoya, J. A. (2006). Multicultural education in the mental health professions: A meta-analytic review. *Journal of Counseling Psychology, 53*, 132–145. doi:10.1037/0022-0167.53.1.132

Snarski, M., Scogin, F., DiNapoli, E., Presnell, A., McAlpine, J., & Marcinak, J. (2011). The effects of behavioral activation therapy with inpatient geriatric psychiatry patients. *Behavior Therapy, 42*, 100–108. doi:10.1016/j.beth.2010.05.001

Steuer, J. L., & Hammen, C. L. (1983). Cognitive-behavioral group therapy for the depressed elderly: Issues and adaptations. *Cognitive Therapy and Research, 7*, 285–296. doi:10.1007/BF01177552

Sue, D. W., & Sue, D. (2003). *Counseling the culturally diverse: Theory and practice* (4th ed.). New York, NY: Wiley.

Sue, S. (1998). In search of cultural competence in psychotherapy and counseling. *American Psychologist, 53*, 440–448. doi:10.1037/0003-066X.53.4.440

Sue, S., Fujino, D. C., Hu, L., Takeuchi, D. T., & Zane, N. W. S. (1991). Community mental health services for ethnic minority groups: A test of the cultural responsiveness hypothesis. *Journal of Consulting and Clinical Psychology, 59*, 533–540. doi:10.1037/0022-006X.59.4.533

Tariq, S. H., Tumosa, N., Chibnall, J. T., Perry, H. M., III, & Morley, J. E. (2006). The Saint Louis University Mental Status (SLUMS) Examination for detecting mild cognitive impairment and dementia is more sensitive than the Mini-Mental Status Examination (MMSE)—A pilot study. *The American Journal of Geriatric Psychiatry, 14*, 900–910. doi:10.1097/01.JGP.0000221510.33817.86

Teri, L., & Lewinsohn, P. (1982). Modification of the Pleasant and Unpleasant Events Schedules for use with the elderly. *Journal of Consulting and Clinical Psychology, 50*, 444–445. doi:10.1037/0022-006X.50.3.444

Teri, L., Logsdon, R. G., Uomoto, J., & McCurry, S. M. (1997). Behavioral treatment of depression in dementia patients: A controlled clinical trial. *The Journals of Gerontology: Series B. Psychological Sciences and Social Sciences, 52*, 159–166. doi:10.1093/geronb/52B.4.P159

Teri, L., & Uomoto, J. M. (1991). Reducing excess disability in dementia patients: Training caregivers to manage patient depression. *Clinical Gerontologist, 10*, 49–63. doi:10.1300/J018v10n04_06

Thompson, L. W. (1996). Cognitive-behavioral therapy and treatment for late life depression. *Journal of Clinical Psychiatry, 57*(Suppl. 5), 29–37.

Thompson, L. W., Coon, D. W., Gallagher-Thompson, D., Sommer, B. R., & Koin, D. (2001). Comparison of desipramine and cognitive/behavioral therapy in the treatment of elderly outpatients with mild-to-moderate depression. *The American Journal of Geriatric Psychiatry, 9,* 225–240. doi:10.1097/00019442-200108000-00006

Thompson, L. W., Dick-Siskin, L., Coon, D. W., Powers, D. V., & Gallagher-Thompson, D. (2009). *Treating late life depression: A cognitive-behavioral therapy approach, workbook (treatments that work).* New York, NY: Oxford University Press.

Thompson, L. W., Gallagher, D., & Breckenridge, J. S. (1987). Comparative effectiveness of psychotherapies for depressed elders. *Journal of Consulting and Clinical Psychology, 55,* 385–390. doi:10.1037/0022-006X.55.3.385

Thompson, L. W., Gallagher-Thompson, D., & Dick, L. P. (1995). *Cognitive-behavioral therapy for late life depression: A therapist manual.* Palo Alto, CA: Older Adult and Family Center, Veterans Affairs Palo Alto Health Care System.

Toporek, R. L., & Pope-Davis, D. B. (2005). Exploring the relationships between multicultural training, racial attitudes, and attributions of poverty among graduate counseling trainees. *Cultural Diversity & Ethnic Minority Psychology, 11,* 259–271. doi:10.1037/1099-9809.11.3.259

Unützer, J., Katon, W., Callahan, C. M., Williams, Jr., Hunkeler, E., Harpole, L., & Langston, C. (2002). Collaborative care management of late-life depression in the primary care setting: A randomized controlled trial. *JAMA, 288,* 2836–2845. doi:10.1001/jama.288.22.2836

Unützer, J., Katon, W., Sullivan, M., & Miranda, J. (1999). Treating depressed older adults in primary care: Narrowing the gap between efficacy and effectiveness. *Milbank Quarterly, 77,* 225–256. doi:10.1111/1468-0009.00132

Yon, A., & Scogin, F. (2008). Behavioral activation as a treatment for geriatric depression. *Clinical Gerontologist, 32,* 91–103. doi:10.1080/07317110802478016

Zeiss, A. M., & Steffen, A. (1996a). Behavioral and cognitive-behavioral treatments: An overview of social learning. In S. H. Zarit & B. G. Knight (Eds.), *A guide to psychotherapy and aging: Effective clinical interventions in a life-stage context* (pp. 35–60). Washington, DC: American Psychological Association. doi:10.1037/10211-001

Zeiss, A. M., & Steffen, A. (1996b). Treatment issues with elderly clients. *Cognitive and Behavioral Practice, 3,* 371–389. doi:10.1016/S1077-7229(96)80024-1

3

INTERPERSONAL PSYCHOTHERAPY FOR LATE-LIFE DEPRESSION

PATRICK J. RAUE AND PATRICIA A. AREÁN

Interpersonal psychotherapy (IPT) is a user-friendly psychotherapy that was developed as a treatment for reducing depressive symptoms no matter what their cause (e.g., genetics, emotional strain, medical disease, pain). As we discuss in this chapter, IPT was developed by Klerman and Weissman for the New Haven–Boston Collaborative Depression Research Project (Klerman, Weissman, Rounsaville, & Chevron, 1984) and was later expanded for older adults with depression (Hinrichsen & Clougherty, 2006). IPT draws on psychodynamic theory and uses specific therapeutic techniques from a variety of approaches, including psychodynamic, supportive, and behavioral therapy. It has been widely studied in older adults with depression and in general is an effective intervention for late-life depression. In this chapter, we review the theoretical underpinnings of IPT, as well as cultural, disability, and cognitive impairment considerations, after introducing our illustrative patient, Susan.

http://dx.doi.org/10.1037/14524-004
Treatment of Late-Life Depression, Anxiety, Trauma, and Substance Abuse, P. A. Areán (Editor)

CASE EXAMPLE

Susan is a 75-year-old woman who was referred by her primary care provider for a differential diagnosis of depression versus cognitive impairment. She came to the initial intake appointment accompanied by her adult daughter. Susan presented as a very highly educated, well-dressed, and prim woman. Assessment revealed a Patient Health Questionnaire–9 Item (PHQ-9; Diez-Quevedo, Rangil, Sanchez-Planell, Kroenke, & Spitzer, 2001) score of 12 (moderate depression), and a Mini-Mental State Exam (MMSE; Folstein, Folstein, & McHugh, 1975) score of 30 (no cognitive impairment). Susan had never been to a mental health clinic before and had no family history of mental illness, with the exception of a mentally ill son, who had passed away several years before the intake visit.

Susan reported that starting therapy was not entirely her idea but that her adult daughter had insisted. Susan reported that she had stopped meeting with friends and attending social and medical appointments, but rather than cancel her appointments, she would simply not show up and later claim she had forgotten. This was the sole reason her daughter and physician had been concerned about her memory. Susan reported that she had been feeling low on energy, had not been enjoying things the way she used to, was sleeping too much, and had limited appetite. Because of this, she reported she was beginning to feel worthless and like a burden to everyone. These symptoms were precipitated by her husband's death 8 months before the intake appointment. Although she indicated that she no longer felt grief over the loss, Susan did miss having someone around to keep her company.

After the interview, we invited Susan's daughter, Debra (age 35), into the meeting to understand her concerns. Debra immediately began to cry and stated she was very worried about her mother but was relieved that her memory seemed to be functioning well. Debra then indicated that she had noted a substantial change in her mother since her father's death, and that while Susan looked put together today, she often stayed in bed all day, ate very little, and would not wear makeup or dress in anything other than a bathrobe, which was very unusual behavior for her mother. Debra then told the intake team that her brother, Susan's son, had schizophrenia and eventually killed himself when he was 21. After the son's funeral, Debra's father told Susan and Debra they were to "get their grief out now" and were forbidden to talk about the son and his death ever again. Susan never cried or mentioned her son after the funeral. During this story, Susan simply nodded her head and showed very little emotion. The intake team explained to Susan that psychotherapy might help her with the loss of not only her husband but also her son. Susan's voice broke and she said, "If you feel I should, I will try it, but frankly, you can't bring back the dead."

THEORETICAL BACKGROUND AND
PRACTICAL APPLICATION TO AGING

IPT is a time-limited treatment (12–16 sessions) focused on improved function and depression remission through the resolution of interpersonal problems. The goal of IPT is to help clients assess the quality of interpersonal relationships and any recent changes in them to see whether a link between the onset of the depression and the perception of change in the client's social roles can be identified. IPT views the psychosocial aspect of depression as having three parts: depressive symptoms, social and interpersonal relationships, and personality. IPT views depression as a function of social stress, social supports, and biological or psychological vulnerabilities. Although many older people experience loss, not all older adults become depressed in reaction to that loss. According to interpersonal theory, when a person is biologically and psychologically resilient, and has ample social supports, that person will experience a normal grief reaction to a loss. However, when a disruption in environmental supports occurs or when deficits in biopsychosocial resiliency exist, then the person is at significant risk for depression. Accordingly, depression can be addressed in a number of ways, either through bolstering the person's resiliency or through bolstering their social supports. In IPT, psychological and social resiliency is the target of treatment. As we discuss in more detail below, treatment focuses on better understanding the interpersonal problem the client is experiencing and creating a link between the problem and the impact it may be having on other interpersonal relationships, and then helps the client develop methods for improving interpersonal interactions. IPT categorizes interpersonal problems into four main problem areas: role transitions, role disputes, unresolved grief reactions, and interpersonal deficits. Below we discuss each and how these areas are expressed in older adults (Miller et al., 2001).

Role transitions are problems that result in a change in societal or family roles. Typical examples are difficulties making the transition from high school to college; challenges around becoming a new mother; and in later life can include retirement, experiencing the last child leave home (or return home), physical limitations from acute or chronic medical problems, moving from one's home of many years to a downsized home, or simply an awareness of declining abilities (including cognitive capabilities).

Role disputes are interpersonal problems that result from disagreements, arguments, or other stressful social interactions with important people. For instance, ongoing arguments over money, marital strife, and parent–child disagreements all qualify as role disputes. Older adults are not exempt from having role dispute problems. Common relationships in which role disputes arise include those with spouses, adult children, grandchildren, bosses, and neighbors, and strained friendships.

Unresolved grief involves the painful adjustment to the death of someone close, be it a child, parent, partner, friend, or mentor. The death of a spouse after many decades of being married can be a very difficult adjustment; on the other hand, compared with younger age groups, octogenarians often have a more accepting view of death in general as the natural endpoint of a long life, as they witness the gradual attrition of their peer group over time. As we stated earlier, older adults with vulnerabilities in their social environment, biologically or psychologically, will have a much harder time adjusting to loss. It is important to note here that nondeath losses from divorce, lost fortunes, house fires, ceasing to drive, loss of sexual potency, or other disabilities are technically considered to be role transitions.

Interpersonal deficits are problems that arise from a client's lifelong challenges to bond with other people. These problems are often the result of more chronic personality deficits, such as poor affect regulation in response to social problems. These problems are felt to be a function of poor attachment style, and the bulk of the work is focused on increasing social skills with the goal of increasing effective social support.

EFFECTIVENESS OF INTERPERSONAL PSYCHOTHERAPY IN LATE-LIFE DEPRESSION

Although IPT is considered an evidence-based treatment for late-life depression, the research on this population is relatively small compared with that for cognitive behavior therapy (see Chapter 2, this volume) and problem-solving treatment and therapy (see Chapter 4). In addition, most of the larger studies have focused on relapse prevention and often evaluate IPT in combination with an antidepressant medication or pill placebo, rather than as a stand-alone intervention (Areán & Cook, 2002). To date, the data suggest that IPT is very effective in treating late-life depression acutely (Miller et al., 2001; Miller, Frank, Cornes, Houck, & Reynolds, 2003; Reynolds, Frank, Perel, et al., 1999) but is not as helpful as a relapse prevention intervention when the older adult has experienced more than one episode of depression (Carreira et al., 2008; Reynolds et al., 2010). Recent studies of IPT in primary medicine focus on younger adults (Grigoriadis & Ravitz, 2007; Krupnick et al., 2008; Van Voorhees et al., 2007). Although there has been only one such study for older adults (Post, Miller, & Schulberg, 2008), the specific effects of IPT have not been evaluated on older primary care patients (Bruce et al., 2004; Schulberg et al., 2007).

PROCESS

IPT is a brief treatment, lasting 12 to 16 sessions. As stated above, the main focus of IPT is to identify the prominent interpersonal challenge, formulate a hypothesis with the patient about the communication and attachment styles contributing to the maintenance of the problem, and determine a strategy for helping the client express his or her needs and gain support.

The first two or three sessions are focused on formulating the interpersonal hypothesis using the Interpersonal Inventory (Krupnick et al., 2008), which focuses on the current interpersonal problems the client is struggling with, collecting information about the problem history, and understanding the client's attachment and communication styles. This assessment is considered critical in setting the focus of therapy but is also considered to be an evolving process. This assessment, coupled with the client's history, is used to develop a therapeutic target. This target is shared and thoroughly vetted with the client to ensure treatment engagement.

When the therapist and client agree to the focus of treatment, the next step is to determine the stage of the problem. For interpersonal disputes, it is important to determine whether the dispute is in the negotiation phase (thus open to solution), at an impasse, or is in dissolution (where no solution is evident). The main goal is to help move the client to a state of negotiation, which is done by attending to the communication style and the client's expectations about the relationship. If an older client is in an argument with his or her children, who would like the client to move into their home, for instance, the therapist will first assess whether the move is at all a possibility. If it is not, then the therapist helps the client give voice to the decision in such a way that the children can hear it. If the move is possible but the client does not want to move into the children's home per se (an impasse), the therapist will help the client move from the impasse into another round of negotiation, so that the client can express his or her desire to move, within certain parameters (Miller et al., 2003).

In cases facing role transition, the focus of treatment is on ambivalent feelings about the transition and bringing to the client's attention the positive and negative reaction he or she is having to that change. If an older person is struggling with retirement, the therapist will first elicit from the client the positive aspects of retirement, while allowing the client to voice the concerns he or she may have about retirement. The goal is to help the client mourn the loss of the old role and develop a balanced view of the old and new roles while encouraging the development of social supports in the new role environment. Therefore, an older person entering retirement may harbor conflicting feelings about retirement, feel excitement about a new stage in life, and miss the responsibilities associated with the old life. The IPT therapist would then encourage the client to discuss his or her feelings regarding the loss of those responsibilities while encouraging him or her to find new responsibilities and to make use of social supports (Parker, Parker, Brotchie, & Stuart, 2006).

When working with clients struggling with grief and loss, an initial step for the therapist is to determine the stage of grief the client is in. *Protest* (disbelief that the person is gone), *despair* (sadness at the loss), and *detachment* (letting go of the lost person) are thought to be the three primary stages, and the IPT therapist's job is to help the client work through these stages toward resolution. The IPT therapist helps the client to understand and articulate their grief and share their grief experience with others in their support circle. Sharing the grief is thought to be critical to help the client move through the loss stages, as this will help the client feel supported and will decrease social isolation while strengthening new attachments. Our illustration case, Susan, is an excellent example of what happens when people are not given the opportunity to voice their grief. Recall that Susan was forbidden to mourn the loss of her son, a loss that is exceedingly painful for a parent to bear. Because her husband did not allow her the opportunity to grieve and share that loss with her friends and family, Susan was never able to move through the grief process, which in the end very much affected how she processed the loss of her husband—as one can imagine, that latter loss was a mix of grief and an inability to process and work through the obvious anger she held toward her husband for not allowing her to process the initial grief. As is discussed below, much of Susan's work centered on sharing her feelings about her husband, and eventually her son, with her daughter and other family members (Levenson et al., 2010).

For interpersonal deficits, now more commonly referred to as *interpersonal sensitivity* (Stuart & Noyes, 2006), the therapeutic process is to help build effective social skills so that the client can develop a stronger and more effective support network. Although clients usually report one of the other interpersonal problem types as the impetus for seeking treatment, the work in therapy with clients who have interpersonal sensitivity is to help them improve their social skills and develop a better support system. This can be particularly challenging for older adults who have had attachment deficits for many decades. However, older adults are capable of change, and sometimes change comes about more easily for them because of the wealth of experience and information they bring to therapy.

The decision to focus on a particular problem area is the result of synthesizing information from the Interpersonal Inventory and the client's history and sharing this information with the client to come to an agreement on the target of therapy. Once that target is specified, the IPT therapist uses two techniques to help the client improve their interpersonal relationships: (a) communication analysis and (b) differentiating content and process affect (Stuart & Noyes, 2006). *Communication analysis* consists of collecting data on the client's communication style using interpersonal incidents. The client is asked to describe the last times he or she encountered the interpersonal problem (e.g., the last time he or she was in an argument), and then therapist and client discuss what was actually said in the encounter and how the client felt. Once the client and therapist identify the causes of the interpersonal problem, they then problem-solve new ways of communicating the client's needs and affect, followed by role-play and practice of these new communication skills. Important in this process is identifying the affect surrounding the interpersonal incident. The IPT therapist helps the client to identify their feelings while discussing the incident in therapy (*process affect*) and the feelings the client experiences outside of the therapy session (*content affect*).

From the beginning of treatment, the IPT therapist makes it clear that this is a short-term therapy that will eventually end. In the last few sessions of IPT, the therapist and client discuss termination issues, because the termination of therapy is likely to be experienced as an interpersonal loss by the client. The IPT therapist will be sure to ask how the client feels about termination and how the client can apply what was learned in treatment to this interpersonal problem. A successful termination is one in which the client can identify his or her feelings and express them in an effective manner.

For those patients with recurrent major depression, it is now clear that maintenance pharmacotherapy may be required for a lifetime to prevent the next episode or to diminish its intensity. Similarly, maintenance psychotherapy with IPT was shown to have protective value even when compared with placebo (Reynolds, Frank, Dew, et al., 1999). A secondary analysis of that study showed that those subjects on placebo whose original IPT focus was interpersonal dispute required monthly maintenance IPT sessions to stay well, compared with those taking placebo who received a brief clinical management session on a monthly basis. Monthly IPT with placebo showed no difference on the rate of recurrence of major depression from clinical management plus placebo if the IPT focus was grief or role transition. For illustration, we refer here only to those subjects assigned to placebo and not active drug therapy (nortriptyline) to detect any potential effect from the psychotherapy alone. These data suggest that in those subjects whose IPT focus was role transition or grief, the issues were likely resolved in the acute phase of IPT where all parties received a combination of nortriptyline and IPT for a minimum of 16 weeks. Those with an IPT focus of interpersonal dispute may have made progress in advocating better for themselves in the acute phase, but when assigned to clinical management and placebo in the maintenance phase, their resolve may have faded over time with a return to prior maladaptive ways of coping such that they again became demoralized and depressed. Those with an acute IPT focus of interpersonal dispute who were assigned to monthly maintenance IPT sessions with the same therapist had the opportunity to review and renew their commitment to continuing on a new path of better self-advocacy with the guidance and confrontation, if necessary, of their IPT therapist such that they were better able to maintain their therapeutic gains and did not succumb to depression as often. Maintenance IPT should thus be considered for those patients who show a focus in IPT of interpersonal dispute as they are at a higher risk for erosion of the therapeutic gains they made in the acute phase of IPT.

CASE EXAMPLE, CONTINUED

Susan's initial sessions focused on narrowing in on the target of treatment. Although it was clear from the intake meeting that grief would likely be a focus of therapy, it was important to also determine whether the target of treatment was grief alone or grief plus interpersonal sensitivity. Susan's history revealed her to be a highly social and high-functioning individual. However, she reported having an aversion to interpersonal conflict and managed this by either capitulating to the other person or, as in the example of her husband, never rocking the boat. Over time, this communication style began to bleed into other important relationships. She began to see how her need to minimize conflict resulted in her having a very superficial relationship with her daughter. She also indicated that she had a difficult time with her son's mental illness because she was powerless to minimize any conflict in the face of his delusional behavior. Over time, she simply withdrew from her son and daughter. Susan also realized in treatment that her tendency to distance herself from conflict resulted in her having superficial relationships with her friends. When her husband died, she felt anxious and uncomfortable when asked by her doctor and her friends how she was coping with her husband's death. Rather than express her discomfort over discussing her feelings, she instead withdrew from her social activities, to the point where she was even unable to call and cancel her appointments, for fear that someone would ask her how she was feeling.

Both Susan and the therapist agreed to focus on resolving her grief and improving her ability to identify her feelings and share them with others. Because of Susan's long-term difficulty in identifying and sharing her feelings, the therapist used a considerable amount of role-play and communication practice to help her begin to open up, first to her daughter and eventually to other family members. Through extensive use of role-play, Susan was eventually able to talk to her daughter about her pain regarding her son's suicide and the death of her husband. She initially had trouble listening to her daughter's pain over both losses, but through analysis of these interpersonal incidents, and practicing ways to communicate effectively with her daughter, in 12 sessions, Susan began to develop a stronger relationship with her daughter.

Near the end of therapy, Susan did express her anxiety about termination, saying to the therapist, "I am afraid I won't be able to keep this up, it's hard for me to talk to other people the way I can talk to you." The therapist and Susan spent 3 weeks talking about the skills she learned and her new-found ability to express herself to those close to her. By the last session, Susan indicated she was ready to move forward. She had reengaged in her social activities and was no longer "forgetting" her appointments. Her PHQ-9 went down to a 3.

CULTURE, DISABILITY, AND COGNITIVE IMPAIRMENT CONSIDERATIONS

IPT has been used in a variety of cultural groups and settings; however, the data are limited on its effects in low-income and ethnic minority older adults. Evidence suggests that IPT is effective for Latinos in primary care medicine (Grote et al., 2009) and African American patients (Parker et al., 2006), with very little in the way of modification. Likewise, there are limited data on the use of IPT in people with disabilities. The assumption, again, is that there is little modification needed for this population, because IPT does not rely on the use of written materials or physical activity. Clearly, adjustments for people who are hearing impaired will be needed, including helping clients with their hearing aids.

With regard to cognitive impairments, substantial modifications do exist for IPT (Miller & Reynolds, 2007). The rationale for adapting IPT for cognitive impairment was based on the tendency for most geriatric research to exclude participants with an MMSE score of 27 or less and on the need for research to begin including a more representative geriatric sample (Miller et al., 2003). The inclusion of some subjects with mild cognitive impairment meant that the researchers had to think about testing a psychotherapy in a sample that included some individuals with cognitive impairment when traditional wisdom dictated that an intact memory for prior session discussions was required to build upon therapeutic gains in order for psychotherapy to be effective. Results indicated that participants with cognitive impairment regard IPT as a pleasant conversation with a concerned individual and that the educational and practical aspects were seen as helpful and validating even if the client could not always recall all the details of prior sessions. The IPT therapist needed to spend a bit more time setting the stage for the ensuing sessions based on prior ones, but when this was done, the clients could grasp the gist of the developing theme. In some cases, the clients with cognitive impairment expressed gratitude for the opportunity to vent about how they felt infantilized or smothered by well-meaning family members (usually by adult children) who assumed they could no longer make any decisions for themselves.

As a result, only two important modifications are needed for older adults with cognitive impairments. The first is the need to accommodate family members in the treatment. We observed that accompanying family members who were waiting for their loved ones to have their IPT session often pulled the IPT therapist aside with a variety of questions or concerns about the problems they were facing, such as obstinacy, role reversals, and noticeable declines in competence. These family members, in essence, had become caregivers, and even though IPT is an individual one-on-one therapy with occasional input from concerned others, it seemed odd not to officially include them in the therapeutic process. The second modification involves the need to educate family and clients about cognitive impairment. In other words, coping for these individuals—who struggled with depression in combination with cognitive impairment—needs to include both issues. Executive dysfunction in particular was often noted to be misinterpreted as something else, such as willful opposition, meanness, indifference, or falling out of love. Extensive education for the caregivers was often required about what was being observed in their loved ones with cognitive impairment, particularly when the patient him- or herself no longer had insight into the issue being discussed.

CONCLUSION

As the baby boomer generation ages, the number of older adults will swell, resulting in a dramatic increase in the need for geriatric experts to care for them. IPT is an ideal treatment modality for a geriatric workforce to improve understanding and facilitate working with aging clients who show features of depression, cognitive impairment, or both. We argue for a new specialty of geriatric care specialist, including individuals trained in IPT techniques with a requisite background in gerontological principles. These individuals would be ideally suited to working in a variety of settings, including primary care offices, long-term-care settings, private offices, and the homes of older people who elect to age in place.

REFERENCES

Areán, P. A., & Cook, B. L. (2002). Psychotherapy and combined psychotherapy/pharmacotherapy for late-life depression. *Biological Psychiatry, 52*, 293–303. doi:10.1016/S0006-3223(02)01371-9

Bruce, M. L., Ten Have, T. R., Reynolds, C. F., III, Katz, I. I., Schulberg, H. C., Mulsant, B. H., . . . Alexopoulos, G. S. (2004). Reducing suicidal ideation and depressive symptoms in depressed older primary care patients: A randomized controlled trial. *JAMA, 291,* 1081–1091. doi:10.1001/jama.291.9.1081

Carreira, K., Miller, M. D., Frank, E., Houck, P. R., Morse, J. Q., Dew, M. A., . . . Reynolds, C. F., III. (2008). A controlled evaluation of monthly maintenance interpersonal psychotherapy in late-life depression with varying levels of cognitive function. *International Journal of Geriatric Psychiatry, 23,* 1110–1113. doi:10.1002/gps.2031

Diez-Quevedo, C., Rangil, T., Sanchez-Planell, L., Kroenke K., & Spitzer R. L. (2001). Validation and utility of the patient health questionnaire in diagnosing mental disorders in 1,003 general hospital Spanish inpatients. *Psychosomatic Medicine, 63,* 679–686.

Folstein, M. F., Folstein, S. E., & McHugh, P. R. (1975). Mini-mental state. A practical method for grading the cognitive state of patients for the clinician. *Journal of Psychiatric Research, 12,* 189–198. doi:10.1016/0022-3956(75)90026-6

Grigoriadis, S., & Ravitz, P. (2007). An approach to interpersonal psychotherapy for postpartum depression: Focusing on interpersonal changes. *Canadian Family Physician, 53,* 1469–1475.

Grote, N. K., Swartz, H. A., Geibel, S. L., Zuckoff, A., Houck, P. R., & Frank, E. (2009). A randomized controlled trial of culturally relevant, brief interpersonal psychotherapy for perinatal depression. *Psychiatric Services, 60,* 313–321. doi:10.1176/appi.ps.60.3.313

Hinrichsen, G. A., & Clougherty, K. F. (2006). *Interpersonal psychotherapy for depressed older adults.* Washington, DC: American Psychological Association. doi:10.1037/11429-000

Klerman, G. L., Weissman, M. M., Rounsaville, B. J., & Chevron, E. S. (1984). *Interpersonal psychotherapy of depression.* Northvale, NJ: Aronson.

Krupnick, J. L., Green, B. L., Stockton, P., Miranda, J., Krause, E., & Mete, M. (2008). Group interpersonal psychotherapy for low-income women with posttraumatic stress disorder. *Psychotherapy Research, 18,* 497–507. doi:10.1080/10503300802183678

Levenson, J. C., Frank, E., Cheng, Y., Rucci, P., Janney, C. A., Houck, P., . . . Fagiolini, A. (2010). Comparative outcomes among the problem areas of interpersonal psychotherapy for depression. *Depression and Anxiety, 27,* 434–440. doi:10.1002/da.20661

Miller, M. D., Cornes, C., Frank, E., Ehrenpreis, L., Silberman, R., Schlernitzauer, M. A., . . . Reynolds, C. F., III. (2001). Interpersonal psychotherapy for late-life depression: Past, present, and future. *The Journal of Psychotherapy Practice and Research, 10,* 231–238.

Miller, M. D., Frank, E., Cornes, C., Houck, P. R., & Reynolds, C. F., III. (2003). The value of maintenance interpersonal psychotherapy (IPT) in older adults with different IPT foci. *The American Journal of Geriatric Psychiatry, 11,* 97–102.

Miller, M. D., & Reynolds, C. F., III. (2007). Expanding the usefulness of interpersonal psychotherapy (IPT) for depressed elders with comorbid cognitive impairment. *International Journal of Geriatric Psychiatry, 22*, 101–105. doi:10.1002/gps.1699

Parker, G., Parker, I., Brotchie, H., & Stuart, S. (2006). Interpersonal psychotherapy for depression? The need to define its ecological niche. *Journal of Affective Disorders, 95*, 1–11. doi:10.1016/j.jad.2006.03.019

Post, E. P., Miller, M. D., & Schulberg, H. C. (2008). Using interpersonal psychotherapy (IPT) to treat depression in older primary care patients. *Geriatrics, 63*, 18–28.

Reynolds, C. F., III, Dew, M. A., Martire, L. M., Miller, M. D., Cyranowski, J. M., Lenze, E., . . . Frank, E. (2010). Treating depression to remission in older adults: A controlled evaluation of combined escitalopram with interpersonal psychotherapy versus escitalopram with depression care management. *International Journal of Geriatric Psychiatry, 25*, 1134–1141. doi:10.1002/gps.2443

Reynolds, C. F., III, Frank, E., Dew, M. A., Houck, P. R., Miller, M., Mazumdar, S., . . . Kupfer, D. J. (1999). Treatment of 70(+)-year-olds with recurrent major depression: Excellent short-term but brittle long-term response. *The American Journal of Geriatric Psychiatry, 7*, 64–69.

Reynolds, C. F., III, Frank, E., Perel, J. M., Imber, S. D., Cornes, C., Miller, M. D., . . . Kupfer, D. J. (1999). Nortriptyline and interpersonal psychotherapy as maintenance therapies for recurrent major depression: A randomized controlled trial in patients older than 59 years. *JAMA, 281*, 39–45. doi:10.1001/jama.281.1.39

Schulberg, H. C., Post, E. P., Raue, P. J., Have, T. T., Miller, M., & Bruce, M. L. (2007). Treating late-life depression with interpersonal psychotherapy in the primary care sector. *International Journal of Geriatric Psychiatry, 22*, 106–114. doi:10.1002/gps.1700

Stuart, S., & Noyes, R., Jr. (2006). Interpersonal psychotherapy for somatizing patients. *Psychotherapy and Psychosomatics, 75*, 209–219. doi:10.1159/000092891

Van Voorhees, B. W., Ellis, J. M., Gollan, J. K., Bell, C. C., Stuart, S. S., Fogel, J., . . . Ford, D. E. (2007). Development and process evaluation of a primary care Internet-based intervention to prevent depression in emerging adults. *Primary Care Companion to the Journal of Clinical Psychiatry, 9*, 346–355. doi:10.4088/PCC.v09n0503

4

PROBLEM-SOLVING TREATMENT FOR LATE-LIFE DEPRESSION

REBECCA M. CRABB AND PATRICIA A. AREÁN

Although problem-solving therapy (PST) is considered a new intervention, it actually has 30 years of research evidence behind it, with the past 20 years focused largely on older adults. There are a number of variations of PST, all with a strong evidence base, and all share the same core features, such as using depressed mood as a cue to address problems, emphasizing setting goals, and creating action plans to achieve those goals.

In this chapter, we provide a brief description of the theoretical background, efficacy, and application of PST, and we offer a case example to illustrate its use with an older client who is depressed. We conclude with a discussion about culture, disability, and cognitive impairment, and how PST can be modified for these clinical features.

http://dx.doi.org/10.1037/14524-005
Treatment of Late-Life Depression, Anxiety, Trauma, and Substance Abuse, P. A. Areán (Editor)

CASE DESCRIPTION

A. M. was a 71-year-old woman with a 35-year history of major depressive disorder, recurrent, severe without psychotic features, who presented to an outpatient geriatric mental clinic with residual symptoms of depressed mood, low energy, and hopelessness following intensive inpatient and partial hospitalization treatment for a major depressive episode. Her most recent episode of depression had begun 6 months after she moved to California from the Midwest, where she had lived for most of her life, to help her son and his partner care for their new baby. Away from her longtime friends and neighbors as well as her usual volunteer activities, A. M. was lonely and disoriented. She was also surprised to find that she and her daughter-in-law disagreed over many aspects of infant care, which was very stressful for her. She began to experience numerous symptoms of depression and anxiety—for example, feeling irritable and restless, sleeping for only 4 hours a night, having decreased appetite, and having a terrible feeling that she was failing her family and they would be better off without her. She stopped going to her son and daughter-in-law's house, began neglecting household and self-care tasks, and spent more and more time isolated in her apartment, pacing the hall and ruminating about how things had gone so wrong. She had frequent thoughts that she would be better off dead, although she did not have a specific plan to end her life. A. M.'s son and primary care physician recognized the crisis, and, with their support, A. M. voluntarily entered an inpatient psychiatric facility for a 30-day course of intensive treatment, where she was prescribed lithium, duloxetine, risperidone, and zolpidem. She then attended another 30 days of partial hospitalization treatment, where she learned emotional regulation and other coping skills in group classes informed by a dialectical behavior therapy (DBT) approach.

When A. M. presented to the outpatient geriatric mental health clinic for evaluation, just before the conclusion of partial hospitalization treatment, she reported that she no longer had thoughts of suicide, was far less agitated, and was able to sleep 7 hours a night. However, she continued to meet diagnostic criteria for major depression, relied on a caregiver to look after household and self-care tasks, and expressed much hopelessness and negativity about her ability to live a satisfying life. Her depressive symptoms were still in the severe range according to the Patient Health Questionnaire–9 Item (PHQ-9; Kroenke, Spitzer, & Williams, 2001; score = 21/30). In addition to ongoing medication management and monthly individual therapy, she was referred to group-format PST to address her persistent symptoms of depression. She agreed that she would give the PST group a try, although she admitted being rather skeptical that PST (or any other therapy) would really help her feel any better.

PROBLEM SOLVING: THEORETICAL BACKGROUND AND PRACTICAL APPLICATION TO AGING

PST is an evidence-based treatment for depression that has its basis in cognitive neuroscience and learned helplessness theories of depression. According to research in cognitive neuroscience, having strong problem-solving skills helps people to achieve their goals. Strong problem-solving skills consist of the ability to perceive a difference between present and desired conditions (i.e., a problem); to focus on a desired outcome or goal that would address the problem; to develop a plan for obtaining the goal, including strategies to overcome obstacles; to implement the plan in spite of obstacles or distractions; and finally to correct the plan in the face of new information that suggests a different course of action. Say, for example, you have had an argument with a friend (the problem) and you would like to resolve this disagreement (the goal). In considering this goal, you determine that there are at least three different ways you could achieve the goal (action planning): call your friend to discuss the disagreement, meet with your friend and an unbiased third party to resolve the disagreement, or wait for your friend to call you. Based on what you know about your friend, and how this person has reacted in the past, you decide to wait for your friend to call you first (action plan selected). However, weeks go by and your friend does not call you (failed plan), and you determine you need to select another strategy to meet your goal, so you decide to call your friend to discuss (adjusted action plan). Before you dial, you become anxious about the outcome (distraction), but you practice what you want to say before the call to reduce the anxiety (focused attention). You have the conversation and it results in a positive outcome (successful plan).

For every action people take, whether it is deciding on what to have for dinner, or resolving a disagreement with a friend, they engage in this process over and over again. However, when any part of this problem-solving process breaks down, people become vulnerable to becoming depressed. According to PST theory, depression could be the result of three different pathways: skills deficits, cognitive overload, and inexperience. Some people may be born with weaker cognitive problem-solving abilities, or problem-solving skill may weaken as a result of cognitive decline in late life (skills deficits). Other people usually have good problem-solving skills, but when faced with multiple life events and stressors that they cannot gain control over, they begin to experience *learned helplessness*, the belief that one cannot effectively find a solution to one's problems, resulting in avoidance and withdrawal from problems (cognitive overload). Sometimes good problem solvers encounter a problem they have no experience with and thus are left unable to set goals or choose strategies to overcome the problem (inexperience). In all three cases, as unresolved problems build up, people experience learned helplessness, resulting in avoidance and withdrawal, as well as other symptoms of depression that in turn worsen problem-solving ability. The goal of PST then is either to strengthen clients' problem-solving skills or to help clients reengage their already strong problem-solving abilities. Depression improves as clients begin to resolve life problems and, more importantly, regain confidence in their ability to do so. Although all psychotherapies teach people to be better problem solvers, PST is a much more direct approach to explicitly instruct people in how to solve problems (Nezu & Perri, 1989).

PST provides a particularly relevant approach to the treatment of late-life depression. PST directly addresses new problems that older clients may not have encountered before and encourages them to draw on life experience to address the problem at hand, as well as offering a concrete set of steps for approaching problems. The intervention has not been greatly modified for older adults, with the exception of taking ample time to socialize older clients to the model and having an understanding of the range of specific problems that older adults are likely to present. Adaptations of PST for older adults with comorbid cognitive impairment include using a greater number of sessions and including family members in the action plans (Kiosses, Teri, Velligan, & Alexopoulos, 2011). PST has also been combined with case management to modify the intervention for homebound older adults and low-income elderly people (Areán, Mackin, et al., 2010). In a study not specific to older adults, Rovner, Casten, Hegel, Leiby, and Tasman (2007) modified PST for people with vision impairment, with the addition of tape recorders to remind clients of the PST steps and record the outcome of action plans.

EFFICACY OF PROBLEM-SOLVING TREATMENT

PST has been widely studied in older adults (Alexopoulos et al., 2011; Areán et al., 1993; Areán, Raue, et al., 2010; Arnaert, Klooster, & Chow, 2007; Choi, Hegel, Marinucci, Sirrianni, & Bruce, 2012; Choi, Hegel, Sirrianni, Marinucci, & Bruce, 2012; Choi, Marti, Bruce, & Hegel, 2013; Choi, Sirey, & Bruce, 2013; Ciechanowski et al., 2004; Fann, Fan, & Unützer, 2009; Fiske, Wetherell, & Gatz, 2009; Harpole et al., 2005; Kasckow et al., 2013; Katon et al., 2006; Lin et al., 2003; Mulsant, 2011; Piboon, Subgranon, Hengudomsub, Wongnam, & Louise Callen, 2012; Schmaling, Williams, Schwartz, Ciechanowski, & LoGerfo, 2008; Stanley et al., 2011; Taveira, Dooley, Cohen, Khatana, & Wu, 2011; van der Aa et al., 2013; Williams et al., 2000; Yochim, MacNeill, & Lichtenberg, 2006). PST has been found to be particularly effective for older adults with medical illnesses and physical disability (Ciechanowski et al., 2004). In one study of people age 60 and older, PST was found to be superior to supportive therapy for older people with early stages of diabetes-related blindness (Rovner & Casten, 2008; Rovner et al., 2007). In a study of 700 primary care patients, Areán, Hegel, Vannoy, Fan, and Unützer (2008) found that four sessions of PST was superior to typical community-based psychotherapy and that treatment gains were maintained over a 2-year period. PST has also been found to be effective for homebound older adults. Choi, Marti, et al. (2013) found that PST delivered by Skype was not only effective in reducing depression but also in ensuring regular attendance to treatment sessions. There is also a strong evidence base for PST for older adults with moderate cognitive impairment. Other studies have found that PST coupled with family involvement effectively reduces depression and improves quality of life (Gellis & Bruce, 2010; Gellis, McGinty, Horowitz, Bruce, & Misener, 2007; Kiosses, Leon, & Areán, 2011). Finally, PST is notable for its success in the treatment of depression in older adults who do not respond to antidepressant medication. In a study of 221 older adults, researchers found PST to be superior to supportive therapy and to have a larger effect size than those found in antidepressant trials (Alexopoulos et al., 2011; Areán, Raue, et al., 2010).

An advantage of PST is that it is easily transported to community settings because providers are not required to have prior psychotherapy training to provide PST. Several studies have demonstrated that medical staff and clinical case managers without extensive backgrounds in psychotherapy can deliver PST effectively (Franke et al., 2007; Unützer et al., 2001). PST was one of the intervention choices in the IMPACT study (Unützer et al., 2002), a national clinical trial of 1,800 older adults in primary care medicine; since the results from IMPACT were published, more than 60 health care organizations in the United States have adopted IMPACT, and more than 200 providers have been trained in PST.

THE PROBLEM-SOLVING PROCESS

All of the various versions of PST share the same intervention principles. PST consists of four to 12 sessions and can be delivered in as little as 30 minutes per session. It is a short-term, goal-directed therapy and requires that clients practice the technique between sessions, using a PST worksheet to solve problems on their own. PST is divided into three stages: (a) psychoeducation about depression and what to expect from treatment; (b) problem-solving skills training; and (c) relapse prevention, which includes a discussion of how to use the PST process for future problems. Although the main goal of treatment is to teach these skills to the client and help him or her overcome depression, the process includes a collaborative therapeutic stance, clinician ability to engage and motivate the client to focus on problems rather than avoid them, and support of the client in his or her recovery from depression.

Part 1: Psychoeducation

The therapist explains the PST theory and research as described above, highlighting that problem solving is a natural set of skills all people have that becomes more difficult to access when they are depressed or overwhelmed, but that they can jump-start these skills by applying problem-solving skills in a systematic way. The therapist often uses a diagram (such as the one in Figure 4.1) to discuss with the client the negative cycle of unresolved life problems, symptoms of depression, and decreased problem-solving ability. Psychoeducational handouts can be used to reinforce and remind clients of in-session discussion (see Exhibit 4.1 for an example). Another tool introduced in the psychoeducation phase is the PHQ-9, a brief measure that maps onto the diagnostic symptoms of depression and that is administered at the beginning of each PST session to track how symptoms change with the PST.

One of the most important tasks of this first stage is discussing clients' expectations for therapy and socializing them to the format of PST. Two common issues that older adults bring to the table are not having any prior experience with therapy and, conversely, having extensive experience with therapy that was supportive, psychodynamic, or psychoanalytic in nature. In the first instance, the therapist may need to address the stigma of seeking mental health care. Many older adults find it reassuring when they are told that PST is largely about reactivating their own capacity to solve problems and resolve issues in their own lives and that the therapy is designed to be time limited and focused on present issues. In the second instance, for clients who have previous experience with open-ended therapy, the therapist may need to reinforce that the focus of PST is not on emotional expression or discussing past

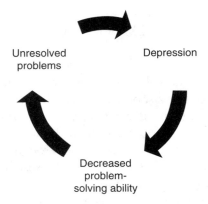

Figure 4.1. Diagram used to explain association among life problems, symptoms of depression, and problem-solving ability. From The Over 60 Program, University of California, San Francisco. Copyright 2011 by The Over 60 Program. Reprinted with permission.

EXHIBIT 4.1
Problem-Solving Treatment (PST)

PST Treatment

- Brief: 4–12 sessions
- Practically focused on current, real-life problems
- Collaborative between client and therapist

How It Works

- Depression is often caused by problems in life
- PST helps clients begin to exert control over the problems in their life
- Regaining control over problems improves mood and helps clients feel better

Depression is very common. It's often caused by problems of living. We all encounter problems in our lives, big and small, every day. It's a normal part of living. Having problems isn't unfair, really; it's just a part of the way life is. If we let problems pile up unresolved, however, it can become overwhelming and lead us to feeling depressed. People who are depressed can learn ways of dealing with these problems. Using problem-solving skills, people can learn to cope better with their problems and feel better as a result.

We can almost always exert some degree of control over our problems. And, if we're able to tackle problems as they arise, it will decrease the likelihood that we become, or stay, depressed. A depressed mood is a signal that there are problems in one's life that need attending to, and we can use this as a cue to take action and to stop and think: What problem might be troubling me? We can then put our problem-solving skills to work and begin to feel better.

Problem-solving is a systematic, common-sense way of sorting out problems and difficulties. If you can learn how to problem solve easily, you can lessen your depressive symptoms and feel better. In PST, the therapist explains the details of the treatment and provides encouragement and support, but the ideas, plans, and action come from you. Problem-solving skills will be useful not only now but can be helpful also when future problems arise.

PST has seven important stages:

1. Write a clear description of one problem to work on. What is the problem about? When does the problem occur? Where? Who is involved? Try to break up complicated problems into several smaller ones and consider each one separately.
2. Set a realistic goal. What would you like to happen? Choose a clear and achievable goal.
3. Brainstorm. List as many solutions as you can think of. Don't rule anything out.
4. Consider the advantages and disadvantages (pros and cons) for each potential solution. What are the benefits of each solution? What are the difficulties or obstacles?
5. Choose the solution that seems best. Which solution seems the most feasible and has the least impact on your time, effort, money, other people's effort, and so on?
6. Develop an action plan. Write down exactly what you will do and when.
7. Review and evaluate your progress. Make needed changes. How has this helped your mood?

Problem solving may not solve all of your difficulties, but it can teach you a better way to deal with them. As you begin to feel more in control of your problems, your mood will feel better too.

Note. From The Over 60 Program, University of California, San Francisco. Copyright 2011 by The Over 60 Program. Reprinted with permission.

events but on actively addressing current problems contributing to depression. It is also important to emphasize that solving problems in between sessions is critical for the therapy to be effective. The initial stage of PST is also the time to figure out whether family should be involved in the client's treatment. For example, older adults with more serious cognitive impairment or physical limitations may find it helpful for family members to be aware of their action plans so they can help support the plan's implementation.

Case Illustration: Psychoeducation

A. M.'s group therapists explained the rationale for treating depression with PST in an individual assessment session before the first group session and again during the first group meeting. She was provided with the informational handout, "Problem-Solving Treatment (PST) for Depression" (see Exhibit 4.1). Her therapists inquired about her previous therapy experience. A. M. reported that she had been in individual therapy at various times in her life, usually where she was expected to talk freely about whatever was on her mind and the therapist listened and provided occasional feedback and interpretations. More recently, however, she had attended the DBT-based skills groups at the partial hospitalization program. Her therapists explained that, like the DBT-based group, the PST group would also involve learning and practicing a set of skills but that the focus would be on finding strategies to better manage the problematic situations contributing to depressed mood rather than learning strategies to cope directly with overwhelming emotions. A. M. expressed her skepticism that PST would be able to help her: "My problem is that I'm no use to anyone anymore—How will you solve that one?" This was an opportunity for the therapists to directly address A. M.'s concerns about PST. They explained that the therapy would help her to start breaking down large, overwhelming, and vaguely defined problems (e.g., "I'm no use to anyone anymore") into smaller, more manageable ones (e.g., "I no longer have a volunteer activity that I enjoy"). A. M. was still not entirely convinced, but she said that she was willing to give the group a try.

Part 2: Skills Training

After the client is socialized to the PST process, the therapist and client work together to create a problem list (see Exhibit 4.2). This exercise is merely a brief review of the goals the client has for different areas of his or her life. Therapists ask about work, health, education (although this may be surprising to some clinicians, many older adults do pursue educational goals; American Council on Education, 2007), family, relationships, legal issues, housing issues, and valued activities. The most challenging part of this process is redirecting the

EXHIBIT 4.2
Problem List

Problems with relationships:	Problems with having a daily pleasant activity:
Problems with work or volunteer activities:	Problems with sexual activity or intimacy:
Problems with money/finances:	Problems with religion or spirituality:
Problems with living arrangements:	Problems with self-image:
Problems with transportation:	Problems with aging:
Problems with health:	Problems with loneliness:

Note. From The Over 60 Program, University of California, San Francisco. Copyright 2011 by The Over 60 Program. Reprinted with permission.

older client to just generate a list of problems. A discussion of goals in an older population often triggers a developmentally appropriate reminiscence process. Sometimes these stories are so compelling that therapists are reluctant to re-direct the client to the task at hand. We recommend letting the client engage in the process, but the therapist must structure it so that session time does not run down and the therapist is able to complete the task in the session. Sometimes generating the problem list can upset those clients with a strong negativity bias. *Negativity bias* is the tendency to pay more attention to negative information than positive information. Clients with this bias can be very distracted by the idea of having unmet goals. When working with older clients with this bias, it is important to check in while the problem list is being assembled and instill in the client hope that these problems will be resolved with time.

After the list is created, the therapist then educates the client about how PST works. The client is first instructed to select a problem from the list that he or she feels is challenging but not so challenging as to be emotionally over-whelming. It is important that the client select the problem for two reasons. First, the client will often know best which problems he or she feels comfort-able working on, more so than observers. Second, allowing the client to select the problem helps the client experience some control and autonomy over his or her life. After the client selects the problem, the therapist then illustrates how problem solving works using a worksheet that includes the following steps: focusing on and defining the problem clearly, setting an achievable goal (something the client can achieve between sessions), creating a list of potential ways of reaching the goal, choosing among goal-directed options for solving the problem, and creating an action plan. After the action plan is created, the client then selects one pleasant activity to engage in that week; activity engagement is meant to be a reward for hard work implementing the action plan. The client is then encouraged to select new problems to work on between sessions, to practice the PST process. The final step of the PST process, evaluating the action plan, occurs at the follow-up session when the therapist and client discuss how the plan went and determine whether the problem has been adequately resolved. If not, as is often the case with complicated problems, they will discuss whether to simply refine the action plan, choose a new solution, or possibly redefine the problem or set a new goal in light of new information. We now illustrate each step using our case as an example.

Problem List

The group therapists instructed the group members on the creation of a problem list during the first group PST session. The therapists invited group members to briefly describe different problems in their life that they would like to resolve or learn to manage differently, and they wrote the problems in point form on the whiteboard in the group room. The therapists themselves even self-disclosed problems that they were working on and added them to the list. Having demonstrated that everyone has problems, the therapists then directed each group member to make a list of problems that he or she would like to begin working on during the course of the group. Group members were instructed either to make a freehand list of problems or to use the worksheet "Problem List" (see Exhibit 4.2) to cue them to problems that may be present in different aspects of life.

Defining the Problem and Setting Goals

A. M. was very quiet during the first two sessions of group PST. The turning point came in the third session, when the therapists and other participants encouraged her to start talking about a problem that was causing her a lot of frustration. A. M. initially defined her selected problem in a very general manner: "I have no energy, I can't do anything." To define the problem in more specific terms, she was asked to give an example of how low energy created problems in her day-to-day life. She stated that she hadn't been getting to the grocery store because it seemed like too much effort and would then get really hungry and order takeout, which she knew was not good for either her physical or financial health. A. M. agreed that this was a concrete, specific problem that she would like to address with the group's support. Her goal, described in behavioral terms and following directly from the problem statement, was to find a way to get groceries that week.

Brainstorming

A. M. was encouraged to make a list of possible solutions that would help her to reach her goal: walk to the grocery store, ask her son to pick up groceries for her, call the grocery store's delivery service, and shop at the corner store. She discounted the first solution as soon as she listed it, "That's no good, that's what I've been trying to do for weeks," and was reminded by the therapists to stick to brainstorming for the time being and that she could evaluate each solution in the next step. In the group format of PST, other group members are invited to offer solutions as well, which can be helpful for the person solving the problem and for the members offering solutions, as it provides a chance to practice problem-solving skills.

Evaluating Alternatives and Choosing a Solution

A. M. was then asked to state the advantages and disadvantages of each possible solution. For example, she listed the pros of walking to grocery store as get exercise, choose whatever she wants, and have free samples. The cons were that she had been trying to do this for weeks, grocery store was a 25-minute walk and she felt discouraged every time she thought of it. For the delivery service, a pro was that she would be able to order nutritious food without having to battle low energy. She recognized that cons were less selection of foods and not getting exercise. She chose calling the delivery service because she felt excited and relieved by the thought and expected that it would take less effort than walking to the store.

Follow-Up

When A. M. returned to the group the next week, she reported that she had applied the solution and it had been a good one for her. She had felt good about having fresh food in the house and had stopped beating herself up for not getting to the grocery store. She reported that she had also worked on another problem on her own over past week, returning e-mails from friends who she had not corresponded with while she was in the hospital. She did not initially recognize her actions as problem solving but was pleased when group members pointed this out and congratulated her.

Part 3: Relapse Prevention

After the client has learned the PST model and practiced applying it to problems in his or her life with the therapist's support, the final stage of PST is relapse prevention. Relapse prevention is addressed in the final session of PST, although it is referred to right from the psychoeducational stage, when it is emphasized that using PST can help both with resolving current depression and preventing future episodes. In a relapse prevention session, the client and clinician will review the client's personal *red flags*, the signs and symptoms that indicate that depression may be returning, along with common problems or situations that trigger depression. A good way to add to this discussion is to review the client's PHQ-9 score with him or her, noting the symptoms that tend to worsen when he or she is overwhelmed. The therapist reminds the client to use depressed mood as a cue to stop and think and realize that there is a problem to solve. The next step of relapse prevention is generating a list of actions that will help prevent depression from worsening, should symptoms return, including using the PST process to address emerging problems. It is extremely important to reinforce the client's use of the systematic problem-solving process to overcome problems and address symptoms of depression. We often find that clients recall elements of specific action plans that were helpful in resolving particular problems (e.g., "I need to talk with Joe when I'm angry about something instead of letting it build up") and have more difficulty recalling, unless prompted, that they can apply the general PST model with any problem. It is helpful to remind clients to use the PST worksheets to address problems when depressed. For a sample worksheet, see Exhibit 4.3.

EXHIBIT 4.3
Problem-Solving Worksheet

PROBLEM-SOLVING WORKSHEET

Name:_____ Date: _____Visit #: _____

Review of progress during previous week:

Rate how Satisfied do you feel with your effort (0–10) (0 = not at all; 10 = Extremely) _____ **Mood (0–10):** _____

1. Problem:_____

_____

2. Goal:_____

_____

3. Solutions:	4. Pros versus Cons (Effort, Time, Money, Emotional Impact, Involving Others)	
a)	a) Pros (+)	a) Cons (-)
b)	b) Pros (+)	b) Cons (-)
c)	c) Pros (+)	c) Cons (-)

EXHIBIT 4.3
Problem-Solving Worksheet   *(Continued)*

d)	d) Pros (+)	d) Cons (-)
e)	e) Pros (+)	e) Cons (-)

5. Choice of Solution: _____

_____

6. Action Plan (Steps to achieve solution):

a)	Task completed? y/n
b)	Task completed? y/n
c)	Task completed? y/n
d)	Task completed? y/n

Pleasant Daily Activities:

Date	Activity	Rate how SATISFIED it made you feel (0 = Not at all; 10 = Extremely)

Note. From The Over 60 Program, University of California, San Francisco. Copyright 2011 by The Over 60 Program. Reprinted with permission.

CASE ILLUSTRATION: RELAPSE PREVENTION

The group therapists used a relapse prevention worksheet to help members record medications (if taken), other treatments, depression warning signs, helpful actions, and a plan for getting help if symptoms were to worsen again and "first aid"/self-care attempts are not successful. Group members were also given the option of continuing on to a PST "graduate" group, a drop-in group that meets every month to reinforce problem-solving skills and provide support. A. M.'s personalized plan included continuing to meet with her psychiatrist and individual therapist, attending the monthly PST group, and keeping extra copies of the PST worksheet handy in a folder in her desk to pull out for the next time she comes across a problem that is overwhelming. She also included in her plan specific actions that would be helpful to her when she is starting to feel depressed, such as sharing a meal with her family, taking a long walk, and reaching out to friends over the telephone.

CONSIDERATIONS FOR CULTURE, DISABILITY, AND COGNITIVE IMPAIRMENT

As stated in the section "Efficacy of Problem-Solving Treatment," PST has been found to be very useful in a variety of cultural groups and among people with physical disabilities and mild to moderate cognitive impairment. Only minor modifications are needed to make PST accessible and acceptable for older adults with these challenges. PST has been translated into a number of common languages, including Spanish, Cantonese/Mandarin, French, Hebrew, Japanese, and most recently, Vietnamese. Although the principles remain the same across translations, the onus is on the clinician to explain the PST stages and concepts in a culturally appropriate way. As an example, in Chinese translations, one important modification has to do with ensuring the therapist retains his or her authority as the doctor. According to Chinese culture, doctors are wise people who have all the answers. If a therapist were to ask an older Chinese client to come up with his or her own solutions to problems, the doctor would lose face, and the client would be unlikely to return to treatment. For this reason, we have modified PST in Chinese to allow the therapist to begin the brainstorming process by offering the client a number of solutions but then giving the client the opportunity to weigh the pros and cons of each solution and then select his or her own (Chu, Huynh, & Areán, 2012). In Spanish, PST maintains the same structure, but there is far less reliance on PST worksheets and forms, as allowing a sense of warm personal connection through informal conversation is important in Latino cultures.

Instead, PST becomes the structure for the therapeutic conversation the client and therapist engage in when solving problems.

As is noted above in the review of PST efficacy, this intervention has been found to be very effective for older adults with disabilities. The main modifications for people with disabilities tend to be on the focus of treatment. Often the problems discussed are those concerning adjustment to disability, coping with frailty, and finding ways to accommodate the disability so that the client's quality of life can be maintained. In the research studies with this population, PST is often accompanied by clinical case management, as some problems often require the help of a social worker who can help the older person navigate the health and social service programs.

The versions of PST that address mild to moderate cognitive impairments tend to focus more on the caregiver than the client. Although the client is actively involved in treatment, the client's caregiver or significant other is often present during the action planning phases of treatment and is there to help the client remember the steps in the action plan. With clients who have milder forms of dementia, action plan implementation can be easily accomplished through the use of environmental prompts and reminders. However, as the impairment progresses, the client will need assistance from others in their environment.

CONCLUSION

Our case study illustrated the application of PST for an older client with severe, treatment-resistant depression. By Session 4 of the group PST sessions, A. M. no longer met criteria for major depression (PHQ-9 score = 1), and by Session 7, she reported no depressive symptoms at all (PHQ-9 score = 0). Her decrease in symptoms corresponded to an improvement in functioning. By the end of the 10 weekly group sessions, A. M. completed all household and self-care tasks independently, had joined a volunteer organization, and reported a renewed interest in activities and relationships. Her functional gains were maintained at 6-, 12-, and 15-month follow-up. Of note, A. M. had been able to discontinue use of two of her medications, duloxetine and risperidone, by the 12-month follow-up.

At 15-month follow-up, A. M. described how her approach to solving problems had changed since going through the PST group. She said that she used to jump right to a solution that may or may not effectively address the problems but now uses overwhelmed mood as a cue to stop and think. A. M. emphasized that social support was an important part of what made the PST group effective for her. She described the camaraderie that developed among group members and people's willingness to help one another solve their problems. The group's therapists reported that A. M., after remaining largely quiet in the first couple of sessions, soon became one of the group's most vocal members and active problem solvers. She readily supported other members and helped them to think about alternative ways to approach problems.

A. M. reported that she had used what she had learned in the group to face new and difficult challenges, most notably a diagnosis of colon cancer. She described how she had used the problem-solving steps to work through a problem related to her illness. In the week after receiving her diagnosis, frightened and still in shock, she considered reaching out to one or more friends who had been through cancer themselves but agonized over whether she wanted to risk upsetting herself or her friends even more by talking about her illness. A. M. reported that the PST process of identifying and weighing her alternatives for action helped her to decide that the possible benefits of seeking support outweighed the potential drawbacks. In the end, she reported that her friends had turned out to be a wonderful source of emotional and informational support.

PST is an effective and acceptable therapy for late-life depression, whether it is delivered in group format, as described here, or individually. Older clients tend to appreciate the approach for being straightforward and focused on resolving current problems. PST is easily adapted when a client is in crisis or when urgent clinical material emerges (e.g., client discloses a past trauma). We teach clinicians to address the crisis, that is, to learn the details of the emerging crisis, assess risk if necessary, and then refocus on problem solving. In fact, the problem-solving process can often be quite helpful in addressing a crisis situation (e.g., a client facing eviction). In this way, the clinician can demonstrate the true utility of PST: not only as something to be used "when you have more time" but also as a process that can be applied in the midst of a difficult situation. PST is not indicated when symptoms other than depression take precedence in treatment (e.g., an individual with bipolar disorder who is having a manic episode or someone experiencing acute symptoms of posttraumatic stress disorder or panic disorder); however, individuals with comorbid anxiety, substance use, and even psychotic disorders can benefit from PST for depression provided other symptoms are well managed first.

REFERENCES

Alexopoulos, G. S., Raue, P. J., Kiosses, D. N., Mackin, R. S., Kanellopoulos, D., McCulloch, C., & Areán, P. A. (2011). Problem-solving therapy and supportive therapy in older adults with major depression and executive dysfunction: effect on disability. *Archives of General Psychiatry, 68,* 33–41. doi:10.1001/archgenpsychiatry.2010.177

American Council on Education. (2007). *Framing new terrain: Older adults and higher education*. Washington, DC: Author.

Areán, P., Hegel, M., Vannoy, S., Fan, M. Y., & Unützer, J. (2008). Effectiveness of problem-solving therapy for older, primary care patients with depression: Results from the IMPACT project. *The Gerontologist, 48,* 311–323. doi:10.1093/geront/48.3.311

Areán, P. A., Mackin, S., Vargas-Dwyer, E., Raue, P., Sirey, J. A., Kanellopoulos, D., & Alexopoulos, G. S. (2010). Treating depression in disabled, low-income elderly: A conceptual model and recommendations for care. *International Journal of Geriatric Psychiatry, 25,* 765–769. doi:10.1002/gps.2556

Areán, P. A., Perri, M. G., Nezu, A. M., Schein, R. L., Christopher, F., & Joseph, T. X. (1993). Comparative effectiveness of social problem-solving therapy and reminiscence therapy as treatments for depression in older adults. *Journal of Consulting and Clinical Psychology, 61,* 1003–1010. doi:10.1037/0022-006X.61.6.1003

Areán, P. A., Raue, P., Mackin, R. S., Kanellopoulos, D., McCulloch, C., & Alexopoulos, G. S. (2010). Problem-solving therapy and supportive therapy in older adults with major depression and executive dysfunction. *The American Journal of Psychiatry, 167,* 1391–1398. doi:10.1176/appi.ajp.2010.09091327

Arnaert, A., Klooster, J., & Chow, V. (2007). Attitudes toward videotelephones: An exploratory study of older adults with depression. *Journal of Gerontological Nursing, 33,* 5–13.

Choi, N. G., Hegel, M. T., Marinucci, M. L., Sirrianni, L., & Bruce, M. L. (2012). Association between participant-identified problems and depression severity in problem-solving therapy for low-income homebound older adults. *International Journal of Geriatric Psychiatry, 27,* 491–499. doi:10.1002/gps.2741

Choi, N. G., Hegel, M. T., Sirrianni, L., Marinucci, M. L., & Bruce, M. L. (2012). Passive coping response to depressive symptoms among low-income homebound older adults: Does it affect depression severity and treatment outcome? *Behaviour Research and Therapy, 50,* 668–674. doi:10.1016/j.brat.2012.07.003

Choi, N. G., Marti, C. N., Bruce, M. L., & Hegel, M. T. (2013). Depression in homebound older adults: Problem-solving therapy and personal and social resourcefulness. *Behavior Therapy, 44,* 489–500. doi:10.1016/j.beth.2013.04.002

Choi, N. G., Sirey, J. A., & Bruce, M. L. (2013). Depression in homebound older adults: Recent advances in screening and psychosocial interventions. *Current Translational Geriatrics and Experimental Gerontology Reports, 2,* 16–23. doi:10.1007/s13670-012-0032-3

Chu, J. P., Huynh, L., & Areán, P. (2012). Cultural adaptation of evidence-based practice utilizing an iterative stakeholder process and theoretical framework: Problem-solving therapy for Chinese older adults. *International Journal of Geriatric Psychiatry, 27,* 97–106. doi:10.1002/gps.2698

Ciechanowski, P., Wagner, E., Schmaling, K., Schwartz, S., Williams, B., Diehr, P., . . . LoGerfo, J. (2004). Community-integrated home-based depression treatment in older adults: A randomized controlled trial. *JAMA, 291,* 1569–1577. doi:10.1001/jama.291.13.1569

Fann, J. R., Fan, M. Y., & Unützer, J. (2009). Improving primary care for older adults with cancer and depression. *Journal of General Internal Medicine, 24*(Suppl. 2), 417–424. doi:10.1007/s11606-009-0999-4

Fiske, A., Wetherell, J. L., & Gatz, M. (2009). Depression in older adults. *Annual Review of Clinical Psychology, 5,* 363–389. doi:10.1146/annurev.clinpsy.032408. 153621

Franke, L. J., van Weel-Baumgarten, E. M., Lucassen, P. L., Beek, M. M., Mynors-Wallis, L., & van Weel, C. (2007). Feasibility of training in problem-solving treatment for general practice registrars. *European Journal of General Practice, 13,* 243–245. doi:10.1080/13814780701814770

Gellis, Z. D., & Bruce, M. L. (2010). Problem-solving therapy for subthreshold depression in home healthcare patients with cardiovascular disease. *The American Journal of Geriatric Psychiatry, 18,* 464–474. doi:10.1097/JGP.0b013e3181 b21442

Gellis, Z. D., McGinty, J., Horowitz, A., Bruce, M. L., & Misener, E. (2007). Problem-solving therapy for late-life depression in home care: A randomized field trial. *The American Journal of Geriatric Psychiatry, 15,* 968–978. doi:10.1097/ JGP.0b013e3180cc2bd7

Harpole, L. H., Williams, J. W., Jr., Olsen, M. K., Stechuchak, K. M., Oddone, E., Callahan, C. M., . . . Unützer, J. (2005). Improving depression outcomes in older adults with comorbid medical illness. *General Hospital Psychiatry, 27,* 4–12. doi:10.1016/j.genhosppsych.2004.09.004

Kasckow, J. W., Karp, J. F., Whyte, E., Butters, M., Brown, C., Begley, A., . . . Reynolds, C. F., III. (2013). Subsyndromal depression and anxiety in older adults: Health-related, functional, cognitive and diagnostic implications. *Journal of Psychiatric Research, 47,* 599–603. doi:10.1016/j.jpsychires.2013.01.017

Katon, W., Unützer, J., Fan, M. Y., Williams, J. W., Jr., Schoenbaum, M., Lin, E. H., & Hunkeler, E. M. (2006). Cost-effectiveness and net benefit of enhanced treatment of depression for older adults with diabetes and depression. *Diabetes Care, 29,* 265–270. doi:10.2337/diacare.29.02.06.dc05-1572

Kiosses, D. N., Leon, A. C., & Areán, P. A. (2011). Psychosocial interventions for late-life major depression: Evidence-based treatments, predictors of treatment outcomes, and moderators of treatment effects. *Psychiatric Clinics of North America, 34,* 377–401, viii. doi:10.1016/j.psc.2011.03.001

Kiosses, D. N., Teri, L., Velligan, D. I., & Alexopoulos, G. S. (2011). A home-delivered intervention for depressed, cognitively impaired, disabled elders. *International Journal of Geriatric Psychiatry, 26,* 256–262. doi:10.1002/gps.2521

Kroenke, K., Spitzer, R. L., & Williams, J. B. (2001). The PHQ-9: Validity of a brief depression severity measure. *Journal of General Internal Medicine, 16,* 606–613. doi:10.1046/j.1525-1497.2001.016009606.x

Lin, E. H., Katon, W., Von Korff, M., Tang, L., Williams, J. W., Jr., Kroenke, K., . . . Investigators, I. (2003). Effect of improving depression care on pain and functional outcomes among older adults with arthritis: A randomized controlled trial. *JAMA, 290,* 2428–2429. doi:10.1001/jama.290.18.2428

Mulsant, B. H. (2011). Problem-solving therapy reduces disability more than supportive therapy in older adults with major depression and executive dysfunction. *Evidence-Based Mental Health, 14,* 77. doi:10.1136/ebmh1175

Nezu, A. M., & Perri, M. G. (1989). Social problem-solving therapy for unipolar depression: An initial dismantling investigation. *Journal of Consulting and Clinical Psychology, 57,* 408–413. doi:10.1037/0022-006X.57.3.408

Piboon, K., Subgranon, R., Hengudomsub, P., Wongnam, P., & Louise Callen, B. (2012). A causal model of depression among older adults in Chon Buri Province, Thailand. *Issues in Mental Health Nursing, 33,* 118–126. doi:10.3109/016 12840.2011.630497

Rovner, B. W., & Casten, R. J. (2008). Preventing late-life depression in age-related macular degeneration. *The American Journal of Geriatric Psychiatry, 16,* 454–459. doi:10.1097/JGP.0b013e31816b7342

Rovner, B. W., Casten, R. J., Hegel, M. T., Leiby, B. E., & Tasman, W. S. (2007). Preventing depression in age-related macular degeneration. *Archives of General Psychiatry, 64,* 886–892. doi:10.1001/archpsyc.64.8.886

Schmaling, K. B., Williams, B., Schwartz, S., Ciechanowski, P., & LoGerfo, J. (2008). The content of behavior therapy for depression demonstrates few associations with treatment outcome among low-income, medically ill older adults. *Behavior Therapy, 39,* 360–365. doi:10.1016/j.beth.2007.10.004

Stanley, M. A., Bush, A. L., Camp, M. E., Jameson, J. P., Phillips, L. L., Barber, C. R., . . . Cully, J. A. (2011). Older adults' preferences for religion/spirituality in treatment for anxiety and depression. *Aging & Mental Health, 15,* 334–343. doi:10.1080/13607863.2010.519326

Taveira, T. H., Dooley, A. G., Cohen, L. B., Khatana, S. A., & Wu, W. C. (2011). Pharmacist-led group medical appointments for the management of Type 2 diabetes with comorbid depression in older adults. *The Annals of Pharmacotherapy, 45,* 1346–1355. doi:10.1345/aph.1Q212

Unützer, J., Katon, W., Callahan, C. M., Williams, J. W., Jr., Hunkeler, E., Harpole, L., . . . Langston, C. (2002). Collaborative care management of late-life depression in the primary care setting: A randomized controlled trial. *JAMA, 288,* 2836–2845. doi:10.1001/jama.288.22.2836

Unützer, J., Katon, W., Williams, J. W., Jr., Callahan, C. M., Harpole, L., Hunkeler, E. M., . . . Langston, C. A. (2001). Improving primary care for depression in late life: The design of a multicenter randomized trial. *Medical Care, 39,* 785–799. doi:10.1097/00005650-200108000-00005

van der Aa, H. P., van Rens, G. H., Comijs, H. C., Bosmans, J. E., Margrain, T. H., & van Nispen, R. M. (2013). Stepped-care to prevent depression and anxiety in visually impaired older adults—Design of a randomised controlled trial. *BMC Psychiatry, 13*, 209. doi:10.1186/1471-244X-13-209

Williams, J. W., Jr., Barrett, J., Oxman, T., Frank, E., Katon, W., Sullivan, M., . . . Sengupta, A. (2000). Treatment of dysthymia and minor depression in primary care: A randomized controlled trial in older adults. *JAMA, 284*, 1519–1526. doi:10.1001/jama.284.12.1519

Yochim, B. P., MacNeill, S. E., & Lichtenberg, P. A. (2006). "Vascular depression" predicts verbal fluency in older adults. *Journal of Clinical and Experimental Neuropsychology, 28*, 495–508. doi:10.1080/13803390590949322

5

EVIDENCE-BASED TREATMENT FOR LATE-LIFE GENERALIZED ANXIETY DISORDER

CATHERINE AYERS, KATRINA STRICKLAND,
AND JULIE LOEBACH WETHERELL

Generalized anxiety disorder (GAD) is characterized by persistent and hard-to-control worry that is often excessive in comparison to the stressor or situation. Individuals with GAD typically worry about routine daily matters, such as health, finances, social situations, and occupational situations. This worry is usually unfounded and interferes with the everyday functioning of the individual, as they are in a constant state of disaster anticipation. Physical symptoms often appear in conjunction with GAD, including fatigue, headache, nausea, sweating, and insomnia, among others (*Diagnostic and Statistical Manual of Mental Disorders*, 5th ed.; American Psychiatric Association, 2013).

GAD is not uncommon in the geriatric population, with rates ranging from 2.8% to 11.2% (Beekman et al., 1998; Chou, Mackenzie, Liang, & Sareen, 2011; Gonçalves, Pachana, & Byrne, 2011; Tolin, Robison, Gartamide,

This chapter was coauthored by an employee of the United States government as part of official duty and is considered to be in the public domain. Any views expressed herein do not necessarily represent the views of the United States government, and the author's participation in the work is not meant to serve as an official endorsement.

http://dx.doi.org/10.1037/14524-006
Treatment of Late-Life Depression, Anxiety, Trauma, and Substance Abuse, P. A. Areán (Editor)

& Blank, 2005). A systematic review of articles published from 1980 to 2007 suggested a broader range, which included higher rates for community samples (1.2%–15%) and clinical settings (1%–28%; Bryant, Jackson, & Ames, 2008). These estimates may not accurately capture disabling anxiety symptoms that are not accurately detected because of confounding comorbid medical conditions and inadequate assessment (Ayers, Sorrell, Thorp, & Wetherell, 2007). Further, many older adults with anxiety symptoms may not recognize them as such (Wetherell et al., 2009), leading to a potential underestimation of GAD.

The symptom presentation of anxiety in older adults may also vary from that of midlife adults who are anxious. Although research in this area is minimal, the few existing studies do support differences in symptom presentation between older and younger adults with GAD (e.g., Diefenbach, Stanley, & Beck, 2001; Flint, 2005).

Diefenbach et al. (2001) focused on worry content in older adults with GAD and found that this population is more concerned with health and family issues than work-related issues, which is the main concern of younger adults with GAD. This is an important finding, given that worry is a distinct characteristic of GAD. Further, Flint (2005) emphasized the difference in somatic complaints, with older adults reporting more somatic symptoms than younger adults.

With these differences in symptom presentation between older and younger adults, it is likely that cases of GAD in older adults are often missed by clinicians. If an older adult presents with a characteristically younger expression of GAD, it would thus seem more likely to be diagnosed, but research does suggest that this is not the case. Although this is a promising start, more conclusive results are required to better characterize the symptom presentation of late-life GAD.

Geriatric anxiety is not only debilitating in itself but it has also been associated with physical conditions and other psychological impairment. Late-life anxiety has been linked with a higher risk for coronary heart disease (Gomez-Caminero et al., 2005; Martens et al., 2010; Roest, Martens, de Jonge, & Denollet, 2010; Roest, Zuidersma, & de Jonge, 2012; Todaro, Shen, Raffa, Tilkemeier, & Niaura, 2007) and substance abuse (Poikolainen, 2000). In addition, geriatric GAD patients experience more somatic symptoms, including gastrointestinal (GI) complaints (Kane, Strohlein, & Harper, 1993), nausea (Haug, Mykletun, & Dahl, 2002), headaches (Zwart et al., 2003), and dizziness (Downton & Andrews, 1990). Furthermore, older adults with GAD have a lower quality of life (Porensky et al., 2009), greater disability (Brenes, Guralnik, & Williamson, 2005), and development of activity limitations (J. Norton et al., 2012) and report worse well-being (de Beurs et al., 1999) than their peers who are nonanxious. Anxiety has also been associated with future diagnosis of dementia in older adults (Burton, Campbell, Jordan, Strauss, & Mallen, 2012). Further, worry symptoms predict early cognitive decline in healthy older adults (Pietrzak et al., 2012). Despite low use of mental health services, older adults who are anxious contend with markedly higher health care costs than comparable older people who are nonanxious (Byers, Areán, & Yaffe, 2012; Vasiliadis et al., 2012).

Depression is often comorbid with anxiety disorders across all age groups (de Graaf, Bijl, & Spijker, 2003; Kessler, Berglund, Demler, Jin, & Merikangas, 2005) and is diagnosed in at least one quarter and possibly nearly half of all older adults with anxiety (Almeida et al., 2012; Beekman et al., 2000; Lenze et al., 2000). With these prevalence rates and implications for physical and psychological well-being, the need for effective treatments for GAD in later life is clear.

This chapter describes the application of evidence-based treatments for an older adult with GAD. The theoretical background to different interventions is discussed, as are cultural, disability, and cognitive impairment considerations.

ASSESSMENT OF LATE-LIFE GENERALIZED ANXIETY DISORDER

Accurate assessment of late-life GAD is pivotal in the evaluation of older adults who present to primary care settings with symptoms that resemble depression or anxiety, as these disorders are commonly seen together (Wolitzky-Taylor, Castriotta, Lenze, Stanley, & Craske, 2010). Frequently used measures for GAD in younger populations have been criticized for use in older GAD populations (Wetherell & Gatz, 2005). One such measure, the State-Trait Anxiety Inventory (STAI; Spielberger, Gorsuch, Lushene, Vagg, & Jacobs, 1983), does not discriminate between depression and anxiety in older adults or in younger populations (Kabacoff, Segal, Hersen, & Van Hasselt, 1997). The STAI is a 40-item self-report questionnaire that contains statements about an individual's current state of anxiety (e.g., "I am worried") and trait anxiety (e.g., "I am a steady person"), which participants must rate on a 4-point Likert scale. State anxiety and trait anxiety statements are scored separately. The trait scale is most often used as an indicator of GAD severity.

The Beck Anxiety Inventory (A. T. Beck, Epstein, Brown, & Steer, 1988) is a 21-item self-report measure that asks individuals to rate statements about their symptoms over the past week on a scale from 0 (not at all) to 3 (I could barely stand it). The total score ranges from 0 to 63, with higher scores indicating more severe anxiety. Although this measure has been used with older adults, its focus on physical symptoms may result in a reduced ability to discriminate between older adults who are anxious and older adults who are medically ill (Wetherell & Gatz, 2005).

The Penn State Worry Questionnaire (PSWQ; Meyer, Miller, Metzger, & Borkovec, 1990) is a 16-item self-report measure that asks about pathological worry to identify those with GAD. Individuals rate statements about worry on a 5-point Likert scale. Some items are reverse-scored. The PSWQ is promising for the use of GAD assessment in older adults, but this population may have difficulty with the measure's reverse-scored items. An eight-item version omitting those items may be better for monitoring the course of GAD during treatment (Hopko et al., 2003).

Another promising self-report scale for GAD is the Generalized Anxiety Disorder 7-Item scale (GAD-7; Spitzer, Kroenke, Williams, & Löwe, 2006). This short measure captures key GAD symptoms and yields both a diagnosis and a score representing severity. Each of the seven statements is rated on a scale of 0 (*not at all*) to 3 (*nearly every day*) on the basis of the individual's experience over the previous 2 weeks. This brief self-report measure has excellent reliability and validity properties, and distinguishes between commonly comorbid depression and GAD.

There are a few age-specific measures of GAD that were explicitly developed for use with geriatric anxiety patients. The Geriatric Anxiety Scale (GAS; Segal, June, Payne, Coolidge, & Yochim, 2010) is a brief, 30-item self-report measure of geriatric anxiety. The measure includes three domains of anxiety symptoms (cognitive, somatic, and affective) and five items of worry content. This measure has demonstrated good internal reliability and good convergent and construct validity in community-dwelling and in clinical samples. The Geriatric Anxiety Inventory (GAI; Pachana et al., 2007) is a 20-item self-report measure that consists of *agree–disagree* statements. The measure does not focus solely on physical symptoms in order to avoid confusion with medical conditions (Pachana et al., 2007). It also exhibits excellent psychometric properties, discriminating well between older adults who are anxious and older adults who are nonanxious.

Clinicians should be aware of several key points when assessing late-life GAD. First, physical symptoms are often overendorsed, while anxious thoughts symptoms are typically underendorsed. This is due to lack of insight that may interfere with the assessment. Thus, clinician-administered measures may be more accurate than self-reports. Finally, older adults may have difficulty with reverse-scored items because such items require intact executive functioning that may not be present in older adults with GAD (Mohlman & Gorman, 2005). Therefore, clinicians should carefully select the measures they use with this population, weighing the pros and cons of each.

CASE ILLUSTRATION: ASSESSMENT

Allen is a 75-year-old Caucasian married man who presented to his primary care physician with complaints of heart palpitations, GI distress, difficulty initiating and maintaining sleep, and persistent worry. Unable to find any medical rationale for his physical symptoms, the physician referred him to a clinical psychologist for further evaluation. Allen was subsequently given a battery of tests, including neurocognitive evaluation, clinical interview, and self-report assessments for anxiety and depression to determine a diagnosis. Results of a brief neurocognitive screen, which included the Repeatable Battery for the Assessment of Neuropsychological Status (Randolph, Tierney, Mohr, & Chase, 1998), indicated mild impairment in executive functioning. Other areas of cognitive functioning were within normal range.

Allen reported notable anxiety symptoms on the GAI (total score = 15; clinically significant range). This self-report questionnaire was chosen for the readability (*agree–disagree* questions) and reliability and validity with older populations who are anxious. During the clinical interview, Allen reported uncontrollable worry, sleeping problems, fatigue, and restlessness. He noted that he could not stop thinking about his son's divorce and reported several other worry domains (housing, his health). Allen's wife noted that he has "always been a worry wart" and that his anxiety seemed to have increased in the past several months.

Although Allen verbally denied feelings of depression, this was somewhat inconsistent with his responses on the Geriatric Depression Scale (total score = 15; mildly depressed range), which is a 30-item self-report measure that requires individuals to answer *yes* or *no* questions to assess for late-life depression (see Yesavage et al., 1983). He was taking Ambien for his sleeping difficulties.

Given his constellation of symptoms, it appeared as though Allen met criteria for GAD. Specifically, Allen reported uncontrollable worry lasting more days than not for at least 6 months. His worry was present most of the time throughout his day. Further, he reported several physical symptoms that increased when he was experiencing worry, such as fatigue, sleeping difficulties, and restlessness. In addition, Allen reported increasing difficulty in everyday activities, such as household chores and errands, because of his uncontrollable worry.

TREATMENTS FOR LATE-LIFE ANXIETY

Several treatments for late-life anxiety are available. These treatments include cognitive behavior therapy (CBT), psychopharmacology, relaxation training, supportive therapy, acceptance and commitment therapy, and problem-solving therapy. In this section, we review the theory and research support for each treatment and provide treatment recommendations for geriatric patients with cognitive impairment.

Cognitive Behavior Therapy

CBT has been the subject of most treatment research on late-life GAD. This set of time-limited treatment techniques aims to identify maladaptive cognitions and restructure them into more realistic thoughts (A. T. Beck, 1964). CBT emphasizes the intimate link between behaviors, emotions, and cognition; when any of these components is irrational or negative, it impacts the other aspects. Thus, CBT works to break this cycle by intervening at the level of thoughts and behaviors, or both simultaneously, to change dysfunctional thinking and thus improve mood and behavior (J. S. Beck, 1995). The CBT model conceptualizes real-life problems in a cognitive framework, showing the patient how his or her distorted thought processes create dysfunctional behaviors and how this pattern is perpetuated (J. S. Beck, 1995). CBT is unique in that it is highly problem-focused, rather than exploratory, and requires the active participation of the patient (J. S. Beck, 1995). Sessions are structured and often take on a didactic feel, with the clinician providing extensive education to the patient about the causes, effects, and perpetuating factors of his or her dysfunctional thoughts (J. S. Beck, 1995). Clinicians work with patients to alter these maladaptive patterns, placing an emphasis on real-world practice so that patients can internalize these techniques and apply them beyond the therapeutic setting.

CBT is effective for geriatric depression (Serfaty et al., 2009), but it is substantially less effective for GAD in older adults than in younger adults (Covin, Ouimet, Seeds, & Dozois, 2008; Wetherell, Petkus, Thorp, et al., 2013). Several studies have examined the use of CBT for late-life GAD (e.g., Stanley, Beck, & Glassco, 1996; Stanley et al., 2003, 2009; Wetherell, Gatz, & Craske, 2003). Although most evidence suggests that CBT is more effective than wait-list, minimal contact, or treatment as usual for GAD in older adults (e.g., Schuurmans et al., 2006; Stanley et al., 2003, 2009, 2014; Wetherell et al., 2003), CBT is no more effective than several other interventions (Stanley et al., 1996; Wetherell et al., 2003). This suggests that what are normally considered the active ingredients of CBT—namely, learning skills to manage thoughts, sensations, and behaviors associated with anxiety—do not provide additional benefits beyond the nonspecific elements of spending time with a therapist and/or a group of same-age peers who are anxious. Under the circumstances, it may be possible to conclude that psychotherapy and/or supportive group contact is helpful but not that CBT per se is effective in treating older adults with GAD.

Two recent meta-analyses (Gonçalves & Byrne, 2012; Gould, Coulson, & Howard, 2012) emphasized the point that on average, CBT is better than nothing for GAD in older people. However, the effect size relative to no treatment is only in the medium range, and when compared with active comparators, including supportive therapy and a (deliberately unsupportive) discussion group, the effect of CBT is small.

In the first randomized trial of CBT for GAD in older adults, Stanley et al. (1996) found comparable effects for a 14-week course of group-administered CBT and a similar course of group supportive therapy in a group of 31 participants at least 55 years of age. Effect sizes were in the large range for both treatments on measures of worry, anxiety, and depression.

Stanley et al. (2003) then examined the use of individually administered CBT with older adults in comparison with a limited contact control group. In this study, CBT consisted of education, awareness, relaxation exercises, cognitive therapy, and gradual exposure, whereas the control group consisted of brief weekly phone calls to discuss symptoms. Older adults (ages 60 and older) were randomly assigned into one of the groups (CBT, $n = 39$; limited contact control, $n = 41$). Treatment lasted a total of 15 weeks, with measures given at pretreatment, midtreatment, and posttreatment intervals. Results revealed benefits of CBT over the limited contact group, although both groups exhibited reduction in symptoms. Further, the treatment outcomes for CBT did not achieve the levels of improvement that younger adults with GAD experience with this intervention.

Stanley et al. (2009) then focused on the use of CBT in primary care settings, where the majority of older adults initially present with anxiety symptoms. The study compared CBT, which uses common techniques such as education, awareness, relaxation, motivational interviewing, cognitive therapy, sleep hygiene, and exposure to enhanced usual care (EUC), which consisted of biweekly supportive phone calls. Adults ages 60 and older were randomized into these two conditions, with 70 in the CBT group and 64 in the EUC group. Results of this study revealed that participants randomized to CBT had a greater reduction in worry and depression symptoms than did participants in the EUC group after 3 months. However, they had no greater reduction in GAD symptoms than did the EUC group, and there were no significant differences between the groups on any measures at 15-month follow-up. In other words, CBT participants had only a partial initial response to treatment, and then they did not maintain their gains relative to individuals who received EUC.

Similarly, Wetherell et al. (2003) found that CBT was comparable to a discussion group intervention in participants with late-life GAD. In a randomized control trial of 75 participants ages 55 or over, results revealed that both CBT and the discussion group were significantly better than a wait-list condition but were comparable to each other. It is of note that participants randomized to the CBT condition in this study reported higher levels of satisfaction with their intervention and perceived more improvement than those in the discussion group condition.

Mohlman et al. (2003) found some support for two enhanced forms of CBT, the first of which focused on problem-solving skills, daily activity structuring, and sleep hygiene, and the second of which consisted of improving memory through teaching strategies. Patients with late-life GAD in both enhanced CBT groups showed improvements over wait-list control groups; in the first enhanced group, GAD patients maintained gains over the control group after 6 months, and in the second enhanced group, GAD patients showed a reduction in worry, anxiety, and overall symptoms compared to the wait-list control group. In a follow-up study, Mohlman and Gorman (2005) found that older adult GAD patients with intact executive function reported a greater reduction in worry and anxiety following enhanced CBT compared with the wait-list control group, as did patients whose executive function improved over the course of treatment. Mohlman (2013) also found that in a sample of 35 older adults with GAD receiving CBT, those whose executive function was either intact or improved during treatment also reported the highest level of worry reduction.

These lackluster findings call into question why CBT for GAD is less effective in older adults than in younger GAD populations (e.g., Butler, Chapman, Forman, & Beck, 2006; Dugas et al., 2010; Linden, Zubraegel, Baer, Franke, & Schlattmann, 2005; P. J. Norton & Price, 2007). It is possible that CBT is much more cognitively demanding than other psychosocial interventions, which may pose a problem in a population in which cognitive resources are limited (Mohlman & Gorman, 2005). It may be more difficult for older adults to learn and implement the many techniques taught in CBT and complete homework assignments between sessions. As such, older adults may not receive all of the benefits that CBT provides to younger populations with GAD.

Other recent research does at least suggest that CBT is not difficult to disseminate among older adults with GAD. For example, supervised lay providers were able to perform CBT with outcomes comparable to trained mental health providers (Calleo et al., 2013; Stanley et al., 2014); telephone delivery was more effective than a wait-list (Brenes, Miller, Williamson, McCall, & Knudson, 2012); and an open-label trial of a computer-based CBT protocol reduced GAD symptom scores in a sample of 22 older adults with anxiety disorders, including 19 with GAD (Zou et al., 2012). As yet, no similar dissemination trials have been conducted using relaxation training or other approaches with older GAD patients.

In summary, although CBT is better than nothing for older adults with GAD, recent studies have found that the efficacy of this treatment is moderate at best (Ayers et al., 2007; Gonçalves & Byrne, 2012; Gould et al., 2012; Hendriks, Oude Voshaar, Keijsers, Hoogduin, & van Balkom, 2008; Stanley et al., 2009; Wetherell et al., 2003). Even when compared with attention control placebos and minimal contact conditions, CBT is still only modestly effective (Ayers et al., 2007; Gonçalves & Byrne, 2012; Gould et al., 2012; Hendriks et al., 2008; Stanley et al., 2009). Because CBT requires considerably more effort on the part of patients (e.g., daily homework assignments to monitor and challenge their thoughts) than do interventions such as supportive therapy, it is probably not the most appropriate first-line treatment for most older adults with GAD.

Psychopharmacology

Older adults are often wary of psychotropic medications because of potential side effects, a preference to limit their medications, and the associated cost (Metge, Grymonpre, Dahl, & Yogendran, 2005; Thorp et al., 2009). Because GAD is associated with both hypervigilance to somatic sensations and worry about negative consequences, it is no surprise that older GAD patients in particular are often very reluctant to take medications for their condition. Similarly, physicians may be hesitant to prescribe medications for anxiety symptoms because of the likelihood of comorbid medical conditions and the potential for dangerous drug interactions. However, medications should not be dismissed, as evidence suggests that psychopharmacological interventions may outperform CBT in the reduction of late-life anxiety symptoms (Pinquart & Duberstein, 2007; Schuurmans et al., 2006, 2009; Wolitzky-Taylor et al., 2010). In addition, older adults may comply with medications for a longer period of time than with psychotherapeutic approaches (Wolitzky-Taylor et al., 2010).

A meta-analysis of 32 studies including 2,484 older adults with anxiety disorders found that the within-subject effects of pharmacotherapy were approximately twice as large, on average, as the effects of behavioral interventions (Pinquart & Duberstein, 2007). The authors noted that individuals receiving pill placebos (the standard control condition in medication studies) typically show more improvement than do individuals assigned to wait-list or other no-treatment conditions (the standard control condition in studies of CBT for late-life GAD). In fact, the average effect size of pill placebo ($d = 1.06$) was larger (albeit not significantly so) than the average effect size of behavioral interventions ($d = 0.81$) for older adults with anxiety. The samples were not restricted to individuals with GAD, the pharmacotherapy category included benzodiazepines, as well as selective serotonin reuptake inhibitors (SSRIs) and other antidepressant and antianxiety medications, and the behavioral interventions category was not limited to CBT. However, despite these limitations, this meta-analysis does suggest that medications may be a more effective and appropriate first-line treatment for geriatric anxiety than psychotherapy.

Only one study has directly compared a medication with CBT in a sample of older adults that included individuals with GAD (Schuurmans et al., 2006). In this investigation, 84 older adults with GAD, panic disorder, agoraphobia, or social phobia were randomly assigned to 15 individual sessions of CBT, sertraline (up to 150 mg/day), or wait-list. Those receiving sertraline showed more improvement on worry symptoms than did individuals who received CBT immediately following treatment and at 3-month follow-up. Effect sizes on measures of worry, anxiety, and depression were in the medium range for CBT and in the large range for sertraline. At 1-year follow-up, sertraline was more effective than CBT on measures of worry and anxiety (Schuurmans et al., 2009). This study is limited by the fact that not all participants were diagnosed with GAD, dropout was high, and the 1-year naturalistic follow-up did not provide information about continuation of care (i.e., whether those in the sertraline condition remained on the drug, what other treatments individuals in both conditions had received).

The results from Gonçalves and Byrne's (2012) more recent meta-analysis are consistent with Schuurmans et al.'s (2006) and Pinquart and Duberstein's (2007) work. Their findings indicate that both SSRI medications and benzodiazepines are more effective, on average, than pill placebo. Although CBT is more effective than wait-list or usual care, it is equivalent to attention placebo and to other forms of psychotherapy. Thus, overall it appears that empirical support for pharmacotherapy is stronger than support for CBT, as a form of treatment distinct from supportive therapy or similar approaches, in older adults with GAD.

It is important to note that not all anxiolytic medications are equivalent. Benzodiazepines (e.g., alprazolam/Xanax, lorazepam/Ativan, diazepam/Valium), although effective, carry risks of falls (Pariente et al., 2008), fractures (Gray et al., 2006), and cognitive impairment (Wright et al., 2009) and are not considered appropriate for long-term (i.e., longer than 6 weeks) use in older individuals. SSRI medications (e.g., citalopram/Celexa, paroxetine/Paxil, sertraline/Zoloft), serotonin and norepinephrine reuptake inhibitor (SNRI) medications (e.g., venlafaxine/Effexor XR), and quetiapine (e.g., Seroquel) are effective for GAD in older adults and generally considered safer than benzodiazepines (Katz, Reynolds, Alexopoulos, & Hackett, 2002; Lenze et al., 2005, 2009; Mezhebovsky, Magi, She, Datto, & Eriksson, 2013). For these reasons, these medications should be considered a first-line treatment for GAD in older adults.

Evidence for medication–psychotherapy combinations to treat late-life GAD is limited. In one investigation, a combination of CBT plus medication management did not appear to reduce worry or anxiety any more than did medication alone (Gorenstein et al., 2005). In a more recent study, a sequence of SSRI medication, followed by the addition of a modular CBT protocol that included relaxation training, cognitive restructuring, and problem-solving skills training reduced symptoms of worry but not somatic symptoms of anxiety relative to continued medication alone (Wetherell, Petkus, White, et al., 2013). Furthermore, those who had received CBT were more likely than those who had not to remain well for 6 months after medications were discontinued (Wetherell, Petkus, White, et al., 2013). Without an active control condition, however, it is not possible to conclude that CBT, as opposed to merely contact with a therapist, enhances response or reduces risk of relapse. Moreover, the 6-month follow-up period after drug discontinuation was too short to evaluate long-term outcomes.

Relaxation Training

Several studies have provided support for the efficacy of relaxation training in reducing anxiety symptoms in older adults (DeBerry, 1981–1982, 1982; DeBerry, Davis, & Reinhard, 1989; Scogin, Rickard, Keith, Wilson, & McElreath, 1992). Relaxation training usually involves muscle relaxation, breathing exercises, imagery, meditation, and education about physical tension and psychological stress (DeBerry, 1981–1982, 1982; DeBerry et al., 1989; Scogin et al., 1992). Individuals engaged in a progressive muscle relaxation condition showed significant reductions in several symptom areas, including headaches, tension, anxiety, and sleep (DeBerry, 1981–1982). These reductions were maintained 10 weeks after the final treatment session. Notably, continual practice of these techniques beyond treatment is important to preserve these improvements. Studies show that relaxation training is more effective in reducing anxiety than wait-list and cognitive therapy (DeBerry et al., 1989; Scogin et al., 1992), and these gains were maintained at 1 year following treatment (Rickard, Scogin, & Keith, 1994). In a meta-analysis (Thorp et al., 2009) of treatments for late-life anxiety, relaxation training was comparable to CBT. In addition, adding a relaxation module to CBT did not reduce anxiety symptoms more than just relaxation training alone. Thus, relaxation training may provide a desirable reduction in anxiety symptoms in older adults without the demanding conditions of CBT.

Mindfulness/Meditation

Mindfulness and meditation-based approaches are not identical to relaxation training, although patients often confuse them. *Mindfulness* is typically conceptualized as a state of present-focused, non-judgmental awareness. Mindfulness is often taught in groups, using protocols like Kabat-Zinn's mindfulness-based stress reduction (MBSR), an eight-session class teaching meditation, yoga, and everyday mindfulness that is widely available and popular with older adults. Our team found preliminary evidence that MBSR may be effective at reducing worry, anxiety, and depression while improving cognitive outcomes such as memory and executive function (cognitive control) in older adults with anxiety disorders or depression and subjective cognitive complaints (Lenze et al., 2014). We are in the process of completing a randomized controlled trial comparing MBSR with health education (active control condition).

Supportive Therapy

Supportive therapy has also been suggested for treatment of geriatric anxiety, and studies show some support for this approach (Sallis, Lichstein, Clarkson, Stalgaitis, & Campbell, 1983; Stanley et al., 1996). This treatment can be applied in an individual therapy or a group therapy setting and typically involves a collection of techniques to reduce the patient's distress and improve well-being. Sallis et al. (1983) found that supportive therapy reduced anxiety more than both CBT and relaxation training; Stanley et al. (1996) found that anxiety, worry, and depression scores were reduced equally in supportive therapy and CBT conditions. Supportive therapy is not as cognitively demanding as CBT and does not require individuals to complete homework assignments between sessions, which may appeal to older adults who want a less intensive and less time-consuming psychotherapeutic experience.

Acceptance and Commitment Therapy

Preliminary evidence for the use of acceptance and commitment therapy (ACT) in older adults with anxiety is promising. In a study comparing ACT with CBT in geriatric anxiety (Wetherell et al., 2011), both interventions reduced symptoms of worry and depression, although the CBT condition had more dropouts than the ACT condition. This may suggest that the demands inherent in CBT may not fit with an older adult population. A treatment such as ACT, which focuses on acceptance rather than challenging thoughts, may be easier to engage in and provide a reduction in symptoms comparable with CBT.

Problem-Solving Therapy

Problem-solving therapy (PST) is considered highly effective for geriatric depression (Alexopoulos et al., 2011; see also Chapter 4, this volume).

This treatment teaches patients to solve their own problems by using a structured format for defining problems, reviewing potential solutions, selecting and then implementing solutions.

Although PST has never been tested as a stand-alone treatment with older adults who are anxious and who have not been diagnosed with depression, there are several reasons to think it might be effective. First, patients with depression and GAD did as well as patients with depression alone in a trial of PST for older adults with major depression and executive dysfunction (Alexopoulos et al., 2011). Second, in a study of older primary care patients with subclinical symptoms of anxiety or depression, a stepped-care intervention including PST was successful in preventing new cases of anxiety disorders or depressive episodes (van't Veer-Tazelaar et al., 2009, 2011). Finally, life problems can lead to or maintain anxiety (Ayers, Petkus, Liu, Patterson, & Wetherell, 2010), and many older adults with GAD experience mild executive function deficits that can interfere with problem solving (Beaudreau & O'Hara, 2009; Mantella et al., 2007). Because PST is highly efficacious in alleviating depressive symptoms in older adults with executive dysfunction, it appears to be worth investigating in older adults with GAD. It was incorporated, along with relaxation training and cognitive restructuring, into a 16-session modular treatment protocol used in a recently published randomized trial (Wetherell, Petkus, White, et al., 2013). The following case illustration is drawn from that protocol.

CASE ILLUSTRATION: TREATMENT

Jennifer is a 67-year-old retired teacher whose husband had died 16 months before she presented for a treatment study investigating CBT as an augmentation and maintenance strategy for older adults with GAD who have made a partial response to escitalopram. She denied symptoms of depression beyond what would be expected in bereavement, but she did endorse chronic levels of worry that had become more severe and debilitating after her husband's death. She also endorsed sleep disturbance, muscle tension, restlessness, and trouble concentrating. She denied irritability and fatigue. Another prominent somatic symptom was GI distress, which she treated with an over-the-counter remedy (Tums) several times a day.

As per the study protocol, Jennifer started with a 10 mg daily dose of escitalopram. She expressed some concerns about taking a medication at the outset and made several telephone calls to study staff, in addition to her regularly scheduled visits with the study psychiatrist and assessor, over the first 2 weeks to discuss possible side effects. In particular, she expressed concern that her GI distress was worse after starting the drug. She was encouraged to take the medication with lunch rather than on an empty stomach and to use Imodium for the next 2 weeks. She reported that her GI symptoms were still present but not incapacitating. After 4 weeks, her anxiety and worry symptoms were slightly improved, leading the study psychiatrist to recommend a dose increase to 20 mg. On this dose, her GI symptoms gradually resolved, and she reported feeling less tense and anxious; however, Jennifer continued to report worries occupying several hours of each day focused on financial issues, her own health, who would care for her if she were seriously ill, and household maintenance tasks that her husband used to perform. After a total of 12 weeks on escitalopram, she began a 16-week course of psychotherapy.

The first two sessions focused on education about anxiety and worry. Jennifer reported that she had "always been a worrier" and expressed surprise that this "wasn't just normal—the way everybody is when they get old." She was able to identify a number of distorted thoughts and problematic behaviors that the therapist conceptualized as potentially suggestive of avoidance. For example, she reported that she had become very active in various community groups following her husband's death and was now serving in several leadership positions. Although she did enjoy some of the activities, she indicated that mostly she was trying to "keep busy" and not stay alone in an empty house. The net result was that she felt stressed by numerous obligations, with insufficient time to take care of important things like paperwork and home maintenance. She readily understood the CBT model involving relationships among thoughts, behaviors, and sensations, and she expressed hope and confidence that treatment would improve her mood and quality of life.

In Session 3, we normally invite a family member or close friend to attend to find out more about the patient's anxiety and its effects and also to provide information about the treatment. Jennifer had no children and no close local friend she wanted to involve in her treatment, but she did consent to have her older sister, who lives on the East Coast, present by telephone. Jennifer's sister confirmed that she had been anxious even in childhood but had been substantially more so since becoming a widow unexpectedly and relatively early. She expressed a willingness to help by calling Jennifer more frequently and checking in with her about the progress of treatment.

Sessions 4 through 6 were devoted to relaxation training. We started with diaphragmatic breathing, helping Jennifer identify a tendency to overbreathe (mildly hyperventilate) using her chest rather than abdominal muscles. She had some difficulty with progressive muscle relaxation, experiencing paradoxical anxiety about whether she was doing it "right." By contrast, she found imagery much easier and more relaxing, so she decided to focus her practice on that form of relaxation training.

Sessions 7 through 9 were devoted to problem-solving skills. Jennifer's main immediate problems were related to the fact that her husband had handled the couple's finances and also most home maintenance tasks before his death. Although Jennifer was paying her bills and had made tax payments, she had filed for an extension and now needed to file a return. She was also concerned about several necessary home repairs. In addition, she worried about what would happen to her as she got older and who would make decisions about her care should she become unable to do so. She described these problems as overwhelming, saying that she felt paralyzed by fear that she would make the wrong decision and bring on an audit by the Internal Revenue Service, get ripped off by dishonest workmen, or end up "abandoned in a nursing home"; she further expressed "disgust" at herself for not being able to do "silly things around the house" and needing to hire someone to do things that her husband used to do easily by himself. Starting with the tax problem, she was able to generate alternatives, but she needed to be prompted frequently by the therapist to avoid evaluating potential solutions until after she had finished brainstorming. Ultimately, she opted to ask a woman who served as treasurer for one of her volunteer organizations, and who was also a certified public accountant, for a referral to a tax preparer. Her success and sense of relief motivated her to work on the more difficult problems of home repairs and planning for her future.

In Sessions 10 through 12, the therapist gently pointed out "needing to do things right" as a theme that Jennifer had brought up several times. Jennifer was able to identify several related cognitive distortions, specifically, catastrophizing and "should" statements. She also recognized that she engaged in fortune telling (e.g., by assuming that workmen would attempt to rip her off because she was an older widow). Using several different techniques, including drawing a pie chart with numerous possible outcomes to challenge overestimations of risk, Jennifer was able to generate more realistic thoughts, but she reported that "although she could think them, she couldn't always make herself believe them."

Because Jennifer had reported sleep disturbance, the therapist spent Session 13 teaching her about sleep hygiene. Jennifer had been spending time in bed engaged in other activities, such as paying bills and using her computer for volunteer work. Afterward, she found it difficult to simply put her laptop on the nightstand, lie down, and go to sleep. As a result, she often engaged in a pattern of trying to get to sleep, watching the clock, and worrying about the consequences of another sleepless night on the next day's activities. Among other behavioral changes, Jennifer began to keep her computer out of the bedroom, working at the kitchen table instead.

The final three sessions were devoted to continued practice and relapse prevention. Jennifer continued to work on problem solving. She began to get estimates for home repairs and asked her niece to serve as her health care power of attorney. She also decided to relinquish some of her volunteer activities in order to reduce her stress level. She found that, contrary to expectations, being alone in her quiet house was peaceful rather than lonely.

Following 16 sessions of therapy, the study team continued to follow Jennifer for another 6 months. During this time, she continued to take pills provided by the research study; neither she nor the study team knew whether she had been randomly assigned to stay on the medication or taper to a pill placebo. She reported no exacerbations of anxiety or worry during this period. At the end of the study, she was seen for a final visit and to break the blind. She expressed relief when it was revealed that she had been on placebo rather than escitalopram. She was happy that she did not need to continue taking a medication and proud that she had developed skills that she hoped would keep her free of excessive anxiety and worry in the future.

Several elements of the description of Jennifer's treatment are instructive. Most important, it is possible for older adults with GAD to experience reductions in their anxiety following treatment. Given the prevalence of GAD in older people and the rapidly growing evidence about its negative effects on health and cognition, the message that this common and deleterious condition can be treated is good news indeed. An SSRI or SNRI medication can be very helpful, but older adults with GAD are often reluctant to take it. We have found that highlighting the health benefits of anxiety reduction (and evidence that among people with hypertension, treating anxiety with medications can reduce their blood pressure), stressing the short-term nature of the proposed medication trial, and providing a great deal of support during initiation and dose changes of pharmacotherapy are essential to ensure that the patient takes an adequate dose for an adequate length of time to experience benefit. Family members can often be enlisted as allies as well. Finally, this process is facilitated by good communication between therapist and prescribing physician. When it is the physician who makes the referral to psychotherapy, this is usually relatively easy; however, because older adults with GAD tend to overuse medical services, even physicians who are less actively involved in the patient's mental health treatment plan may be happy to collaborate in a process that will result in fewer anxiety-driven office visits or referrals to medical specialists (e.g., cardiology, gastroenterology).

With respect to treatment elements, relaxation training is well tolerated and often very effective. We usually teach three forms of relaxation: diaphragmatic breathing, progressive muscle relaxation, and imagery. As was the case with Jennifer, patients usually find at least one of these beneficial. Problem-solving skills training is often quite helpful with older GAD patients, many of whom either procrastinate (like Jennifer) or react impulsively when faced with difficult problems. Cognitive restructuring is not, in our experience, as helpful as other techniques with older GAD patients. Unlike some of our patients, Jennifer was able to carry out the exercises, but she found it difficult to "believe" the alternative thoughts she was able to generate. Other treatment modules that can be helpful depending on the patient's particular symptoms or situation, and that were tested in our trial, were family psychoeducation (included but probably less helpful in Jennifer's case than for some other patients), sleep hygiene (helpful), behavioral activation (for those with current or recent past history of depression; unnecessary for Jennifer), and exposure therapy (for those with comorbid anxiety disorders; again, unnecessary for Jennifer).

CULTURE, DISABILITY, AND COGNITIVE IMPAIRMENT CONSIDERATIONS

Most research on older adults with GAD has been done in culturally heterogeneous Caucasian samples in the United States, the Netherlands, and Australia. Thus, relatively little is known about the ways in which older adults from other cultural backgrounds express anxiety or respond to treatment. In a very preliminary study on this topic, our team conducted a mixed methods investigation with 25 older Spanish-speaking Mexican Americans living in the Central Valley of California who responded to flyers at a mental health clinic, senior center, or primary care clinic soliciting individuals who feel "tense" or "down" (Letamendi et al., 2013). Sixty-eight percent met criteria for a *Diagnostic and Statistical Manual of Mental Disorders* (4th ed.; American Psychiatric Association, 1994) diagnosis, most typically GAD or major depression; rates of comorbidity were high. In this sample, with very low levels of formal education (4 years, on average) and low Anglo acculturation, neither of these factors was associated with anxiety or depression. Most, but not all, participants used Western idioms of distress. Perhaps most significantly, three of the four most commonly mentioned sources of potential help for psychiatric symptoms were not formal mental health services: activities/hobbies, spirituality, and social support were named, along with group therapy. In contrast to prevalent beliefs about the positive value of *familism* among Mexican Americans, the most common barriers to seeking treatment were actually family related, such as perceptions of being misunderstood or rejected by family members.

Cognitive functioning is an important factor in treating older adult populations, as low cognitive function can serve as a treatment barrier (Mohlman & Gorman, 2005). Research has shown that older adults with anxiety have more cognitive impairment than do healthy peers (Beaudreau

& O'Hara, 2008; Schultz, Moser, Bishop, & Ellingrod, 2005), including more impairment in short-term memory (Mantella et al., 2007). Further, older adults commonly exhibit executive dysfunction and frontal lobe atrophy, both of which have a profound impact on treatment response (Mohlman & Gorman, 2005).

As previously mentioned, CBT requires a significant amount of cognitive resources to fully engage in and benefit from the treatment course, which perhaps explains why older adults do not respond as well as younger adults (Mohlman & Gorman, 2005). For example, common CBT techniques require patients to keep self-monitor logs, logically restructure maladaptive thoughts, generate alternative healthy thoughts, and plan individual exposure practice (Mohlman & Gorman, 2005). Each of these techniques requires the use of higher order cognitive skills that may be impaired because of organic factors, thereby placing older adults at a disadvantage in treatment response. Accordingly, Mohlman and Gorman (2005) found that older adults with GAD and executive deficits did not respond to CBT; however, older adults with GAD and intact executive function responded better. Further, participants whose executive skills improved throughout treatment had better posttreatment response than those whose deficits remained impaired. Older adults who experienced executive dysfunction responded equally to CBT and a wait-list condition.

Given the frequency of memory impairment and executive dysfunction, older adults may forget to complete homework between sessions or have trouble relating the more abstract components of this treatment to their own condition. As such, relaxation training is the preferred first-line behavioral treatment strategy for older adults who are anxious and refuse to consider psychotropic medications. Once medications are started, a modified CBT protocol that takes into account potential cognitive impairment and focuses on more personally relevant techniques may be more beneficial to older adults who are anxious. Thus, therapists can implement between-session reminders to complete homework (e.g., phone calls, memory aids), frequent concept reviews (e.g., beginning each session with a review of the previous week's session), and simpler explanations for a technique's rationale. In addition, an emphasis on behavioral techniques (e.g., sleep hygiene, time management, in vivo exposures) may be more effective for older adults than techniques that are cognitively demanding (e.g., self-monitoring, thought challenging).

Clinicians working with older adults should consider the unique properties of this population. A few basic adjustments can be made. First, involving family members and caregivers in treatment planning may increase patient adherence. Home visits, if possible, can circumvent issues with transportation and medical conditions, which make mobility difficult for many older adults. Finally, shortening treatment sessions can remedy problems related to low stamina.

Psychiatric comorbidities are also of concern with treatment of older adults. Several studies have shown that comorbid diagnoses of depression are common with geriatric anxiety (Almeida et al., 2012; Beekman et al., 2000; Lenze et al., 2000; Schaub & Linden, 2000; van Balkom et al., 2000). Furthermore, one study revealed that depression is the most common comorbid disorder in older adults with anxiety (Cairney, Corna, & Velhuizen, 2008). Notably, depression in older adults is associated with more severe anxiety (Hopko, Bourland, & Stanley, 2000), and the presence of anxiety in older adults, regardless of severity, is associated with a higher suicide risk (Lenze et al., 2000).

The prevalence of comorbid anxiety and depression in older adults can have important treatment implications. Psychotherapy is effective for geriatric depression, even among cognitively impaired individuals (Areán et al., 2010; Kiosses, Teri, Velligan, Alexopoulos, 2011; Pinquart, Duberstein, & Lyness, 2006; Serfaty et al., 2009); we have found that older adults who are both depressed and anxious are more likely to respond to psychotherapy than are older adults with anxiety alone (Wuthrich & Rapee, 2013). However, psychotherapeutic interventions may take longer to improve symptoms if both anxiety and depression are present in older adults.

Many older adults have complex medical histories, which can also affect anxiety disorders (Dawson, Kline, Wiancko, & Wells, 1986; Haley, 1996), and those with geriatric anxiety may have an even more complicated medical picture. Perhaps the most salient health risk related to geriatric anxiety is cardiovascular disease, which is associated with higher mortality rates in older adults who are anxious (Roest et al., 2012; Smoller, Pollack, Wassertheil-Smoller, 2007). Chest pain and other cardiac symptoms are commonly seen in older adults who are anxious (Goldberg, Morris, & Christian, 1990). In addition to cardiac problems, respiratory disorders (Vögele & von Luepoldt, 2008) and vestibular symptoms (Downton & Andrews, 1990) are also common comorbidities. With the prevalence of these comorbidities, accurate diagnosis of older adults presenting with these symptoms can be difficult, as anxiety-related symptoms can be mistaken for medical conditions and vice versa.

In summary, understanding the unique aspects of geriatric anxiety can improve diagnosis, treatment planning and delivery, and outcomes. Communication among treatment providers is vital for successful intervention with older adults who are anxious. Medical comorbidities can convolute the symptom picture, and thus a medical differential diagnosis is often indicated for older adults. Contact with the primary care physician can be helpful in providing a complete diagnostic picture.

CONCLUSION

With the geriatric population increasing exponentially, it is imperative for clinicians to become proficient in the assessment and treatment of older adults who are anxious. Working with this population is marked by numerous challenges, including differences in symptom presentation, medication responsiveness, psychiatric comorbidities, treatment efficacy, cognitive capacity, physical ability, and health status. Further, empirical research highlighting these differences and providing more accurate clinical information is lacking, leaving clinicians to use potentially ineffective assessment techniques and treatment interventions. However, many well-known interventions can be tailored to maximize the strengths and minimize the weaknesses of the older adult population. It is important to note that every older adult will present with unique experiences and strengths, and thus an individualized assessment and treatment approach is vital to an effective intervention.

REFERENCES

Alexopoulos, G. S., Raue, P. J., Kiosses, D. N., Mackin, R., Kanellopoulos, D., McCulloch, C., & Areán, P. A. (2011). Problem-solving therapy and supportive therapy in older adults with major depression and executive dysfunction. *Archives of General Psychiatry, 68*, 33–41. doi:10.1001/archgenpsychiatry.2010.177

Almeida, O., Draper, B., Pirkis, J., Snowdon, J., Lautenschlager, N., Byrne, G., & . . . Pfaff, J. (2012). Anxiety, depression, and comorbid anxiety and depression: Risk factors and outcome over two years. *International Psychogeriatrics/IPA, 24*, 1622–1632. doi:10.1017/S104161021200107X.

American Psychiatric Association. (1994). *Diagnostic and statistical manual of mental disorders* (4th ed.). Washington, DC: Author.

American Psychiatric Association. (2013). *Diagnostic and statistical manual of mental disorders* (5th ed.). Washington, DC: Author.

Areán, P. A., Raue, P., Mackin, R., Kanellopoulos, D., McCulloch, C., & Alexopoulos, G. S. (2010). Problem-solving therapy and supportive therapy in older adults with major depression and executive dysfunction. *The American Journal of Psychiatry, 167*, 1391–1398. doi:10.1176/appi.ajp.2010.09091327

Ayers, C. R., Petkus, A., Liu, L., Patterson, T. L., & Wetherell, J. L. (2010). Negative life events and avoidant coping are associated with poorer long-term outcome in older adults treated for generalized anxiety disorder. *Journal of Experimental Psychopathology, 1*, 146–154. doi:10.5127/jep.003110

Ayers, C. R., Sorrell, J. T., Thorp, S. R., & Wetherell, J. L. (2007). Evidence-based psychological treatments for late-life anxiety. *Psychology and Aging, 22*, 8–17. doi:10.1037/0882-7974.22.1.8

Beaudreau, S. A., & O'Hara, R. (2008). Late-life anxiety and cognitive impairment: A review. *The American Journal of Geriatric Psychiatry, 16*, 790–803. doi:10.1097/JGP.0b013e31817945c3

Beaudreau, S. A., & O'Hara, R. (2009). The association of anxiety and depressive symptoms with cognitive performance in community-dwelling older adults. *Psychology and Aging, 24*, 507–512. doi:10.1037/a0016035

Beck, A. T. (1964). Thinking and depression: II. Theory and therapy. *Archives of General Psychiatry, 10*, 561–571. doi:10.1001/archpsyc.1964.01720240015003

Beck, A. T., Epstein, N., Brown, G., & Steer, R. A. (1988). An inventory for measuring clinical anxiety: Psychometric properties. *Journal of Consulting and Clinical Psychology, 56*, 893–897. doi:10.1037/0022-006X.56.6.893

Beck, J. S. (1995). *Cognitive therapy: Basics and beyond.* New York, NY: Guilford Press.

Beekman, A. T., Bremmer, M. A., Deeg, D. J., van Balkom, A. J., Smit, J. H., de Beurs, E., . . . van Tilburg, W. (1998). Anxiety disorders in later life: A report from the Longitudinal Aging Study Amsterdam. *International Journal of Geriatric Psychiatry, 13*, 717–726. doi:10.1002/(SICI)1099-1166 (1998100)13:10<717::AID-GPS857>3.0.CO;2-M

Beekman, A. T., De Beurs, E., van Balkom, A. M., Deeg, D. H., Van Dyck, R., & Van Tilburg, W. (2000). Anxiety and depression in later life: Co-occurrence and communality of risk factors. *The American Journal of Psychiatry, 157*, 89–95.

Brenes, G. A., Guralnik, J. M., & Williamson, J. D. (2005). Correlates of anxiety symptoms in physically disabled older women. *The American Journal of Geriatric Psychiatry, 13*, 15–22. doi:10.1097/00019442-200501000-00004

Brenes, G. A., Miller, M. E., Williamson, J. D., McCall, W. V., & Knudson, M. (2012). A randomized controlled trial of telephone-delivered cognitive-behavioral therapy for late-life anxiety disorders. *The American Journal of Geriatric Psychiatry, 20*, 707–716. doi:10.1097/JGP.0b013e31822ccd3e

Bryant, C., Jackson, H., & Ames, D. (2008). The prevalence of anxiety in older adults: Methodological issues and a review of the literature. *Journal of Affective Disorders, 109*, 233–250. doi:10.1016/j.jad.2007.11.008

Burton, C., Campbell, P., Jordan, K., Strauss, V., & Mallen, C. (2012). The association of anxiety and depression with future dementia diagnosis: A case-control study in primary care. *Family Practice.* Advance online publication. doi:10.1093/fampra/cms044

Butler, A. C., Chapman, J. E., Forman, E. M., & Beck, A. T. (2006). The empirical status of cognitive-behavioral therapy: A review of meta-analyses. *Clinical Psychology Review, 26*, 17–31. doi:10.1016/j.cpr.2005.07.003

Byers, A. L., Areán, P. A., & Yaffe, K. (2012). Low use of mental health services among older Americans with mood and anxiety disorders. *Psychiatric Services, 63*, 66–72. doi:10.1176/appi.ps.201100121

Cairney, J., Corna, L. M., & Velhuizen, S. (2008). Comorbid depression and anxiety in later life: Patterns of association, subjective wellbeing, and impairment.

The American Journal of Geriatric Psychiatry, 16, 201–208. doi:10.1097/01.JGP.0000300627.93523.c8

Calleo, J. S., Bush, A. L., Cully, J. A., Wilson, N. L., Kraus-Schuman, C., Rhoades, H. M., . . . Stanley, M. A. (2013). Treating late-life generalized anxiety disorder in primary care: An effectiveness pilot study. *Journal of Nervous and Mental Disease, 201*, 414–420. doi:10.1097/NMD.0b013e31828e0fd6

Chou, K. L., Mackenzie, C. S., Liang, K., & Sareen, J. (2011). Three-year incidence and predictors of first-onset of *DSM–IV* mood, anxiety, and substance use disorders in older adults: Results from Wave 2 of the National Epidemiologic Survey on Alcohol and Related Conditions. *Journal of Clinical Psychiatry, 72*, 144–155. doi:10.4088/JCP.09m05618gry

Covin, R., Ouimet, A. J., Seeds, P. M., & Dozois, D. A. (2008). A meta-analysis of CBT for pathological worry among clients with GAD. *Journal of Anxiety Disorders, 22*, 108–116. doi:10.1016/j.janxdis.2007.01.002

Dawson, P., Kline, K., Wiancko, D. C., & Wells, D. (1986). Preventing excess disability in patients with Alzheimer's disease. *Geriatric Nursing, 7*, 298–301. doi:10.1016/S0197-4572(86)80158-6

DeBerry, S. (1981–1982). An evaluation of progressive muscle relaxation on stress related symptoms in a geriatric population. *International Journal of Aging and Human Development, 14*, 255–269. doi:10.2190/5C1R-9D61-YG2N-A7LV

DeBerry, S. (1982). The effects of meditation–relaxation on anxiety and depression in a geriatric population. *Psychotherapy: Theory, Research, & Practice, 19*, 512–521. doi:10.1037/h0088465

DeBerry, S., Davis, S., & Reinhard, K. E. (1989). A comparison of meditation–relaxation and cognitive/behavioral techniques for reducing anxiety and depression in a geriatric population. *Journal of Geriatric Psychiatry, 22*, 231–247.

de Beurs, E., Beekman, A. T. F., van Balkom, A. M., Deeg, D. H., Van Dyck, R., & Van Tilburg, W. (1999). Consequences of anxiety in older persons: Its effect on disability, well-being, and use of health services. *Psychological Medicine, 29*, 583–593. doi:10.1017/S0033291799008351

de Graaf, R., Bijl, R. V., & Spijker, J. (2003). Temporal sequencing of lifetime mood disorders in relation to comorbid anxiety and substance use disorders. *Social Psychiatry and Psychiatric Epidemiology, 38*, 1–11. doi:10.1007/s00127-003-0597-4

Diefenbach, G. J., Stanley, M. A., & Beck, J. G. (2001). Worry content reported by older adults with and without generalized anxiety disorder. *Aging & Mental Health, 5*, 269–274. doi:10.1080/13607860120065069

Downton, J. H., & Andrews, K. (1990). Postural disturbance and psychological symptoms amongst elderly people living at home. *International Journal of Geriatric Psychiatry, 5*, 93–98. doi:10.1002/gps.930050206

Dugas, M. J., Brillon, P., Savard, P., Turcotte, J., Gaudet, A., Ladouceur, R., . . . Gervais, N. J. (2010). A randomized clinical trial of cognitive-behavioral therapy and applied relaxation for adults with generalized anxiety disorder. *Behavior Therapy, 41*, 46–58. doi:10.1016/j.beth.2008.12.004

Flint, A. J. (2005). Anxiety and its disorders in late life: Moving the field forward. *The American Journal of Geriatric Psychiatry, 13*, 3–6. doi:10.1097/00019442-200501000-00002

Goldberg, R., Morris, P., & Christian, F. (1990). Panic disorder in cardiac outpatients. *Psychosomatics, 31*, 168–173. doi:10.1016/S0033-3182(90)72190-1

Gomez-Caminero, A., Blumentals, W. A., Russo, L. J., Brown, R. R., Castilla, M. L., & Castilla, R. (2005). Does panic disorder increase the risk of coronary heart disease? A cohort study of a national managed care database. *Psychosomatic Medicine, 67*, 688–691. doi:10.1097/01.psy.0000174169.14227.1f

Gonçalves, D. C., & Byrne, G. J. (2012). Interventions for generalized anxiety disorder in older adults: Systematic review and meta-analysis. *Journal of Anxiety Disorders, 26*, 1–11. doi:10.1016/j.janxdis.2011.08.010

Gonçalves, D. C., Pachana, N. A., & Byrne, G. J. (2011). Prevalence and correlates of generalized anxiety disorder among older adults in the Australian National Survey of Mental Health and Well-Being. *Journal of Affective Disorders, 132*, 223–230. doi:10.1016/j.jad.2011.02.023

Gorenstein, E. E., Kleber, M. S., Mohlman, J., DeJesus, M., Gorman, J. M., & Papp, L. A. (2005). Cognitive-behavioral therapy for management of anxiety and medication taper in older adults. *The American Journal of Geriatric Psychiatry, 13*, 901–909. doi:10.1176/appi.ajgp.13.10.901

Gould, R. L., Coulson, M. C., & Howard, R. J. (2012). Efficacy of cognitive behavioral therapy for anxiety disorders in older people: A meta-analysis and meta-regression of randomized controlled trials. *Journal of the American Geriatrics Society, 60*, 218–229. doi:10.1111/j.1532-5415.2011.03824.x

Gray, S. L., LaCroix, A. Z., Hanlon, J. T., Penninx, B. H., Blough, D. K., Leveille, S. G., . . . Buchner, D. M. (2006). Benzodiazepine use and physical disability in community-dwelling older adults. *Journal of the American Geriatrics Society, 54*, 224–230. doi:10.1111/j.1532-5415.2005.00571.x

Haley, W. E. (1996). The medical context of psychotherapy with the elderly. In S. H. Zarit & B. G. Knight (Eds.), *A guide to psychotherapy and aging: Effective clinical interventions in a life-stage context* (pp. 221–239). Washington, DC: American Psychological Association. doi:10.1037/10211-008

Haug, T. T., Mykletun, A., & Dahl, A. A. (2002). Are anxiety and depression related to gastrointestinal symptoms in the general population? *Scandinavian Journal of Gastroenterology, 37*, 294–298. doi:10.1080/003655202317284192

Hendriks, G. J., Oude Voshaar, R. C., Keijsers, G. P. J., Hoogduin, C. A. L., & van Balkom, A. J. (2008). Cognitive-behavioural therapy for late-life anxiety disorders: A systematic review and meta-analysis. *Acta Psychiatrica Scandinavica, 117*, 403–411. doi:10.1111/j.1600-0447.2008.01190.x

Hopko, D. R., Bourland, S. L., & Stanley, M. A. (2000). Generalized anxiety disorder in older adults: Examining the relation between clinician severity rating and patient self report measures. *Depression and Anxiety, 12*, 217–225. doi:10.1002/1520-6394(2000)12:4<217::AID-DA5>3.0.CO;2-6

Hopko, D. R., Stanley, M. A., Reas, D. L., Wetherell, J. L., Beck, J. G., Novy, D. M., & Averill, P. M. (2003). Assessing worry in older adults: Confirmatory factor analysis of the Penn State Worry Questionnaire and psychometric properties of an abbreviated model. *Psychological Assessment, 15,* 173–183. doi:10.1037/1040-3590.15.2.173

Kabacoff, R. I., Segal, D. L., Hersen, M., & Van Hasselt, V. B. (1997). Psychometric properties and diagnostic utility of the Beck Anxiety Inventory and the State–Trait Anxiety Inventory with older adult psychiatric outpatients. *Journal of Anxiety Disorders, 11,* 33–47. doi:10.1016/S0887-6185(96)00033-3

Kane, F. J., Strohlein, J., & Harper, R. G. (1993). Nonulcer dyspepsia associated with psychiatric disorder. *Southern Medical Journal, 86,* 641–646. doi:10.1097/00007611-199306000-00010

Katz, I. R., Reynolds, C. F., Alexopoulos, G. S., & Hackett, D. (2002). Venlafaxine ER as a treatment for generalized anxiety disorder in older adults: Pooled analysis of five randomized placebo-controlled clinical trials. *Journal of the American Geriatrics Society, 50,* 18–25. doi:10.1046/j.1532-5415.2002.50003.x

Kessler, R. C., Berglund, P., Demler, O., Jin, R., & Merikangas, K. R. (2005). Lifetime prevalence and age-of-onset distributions of *DSM–IV* disorders in the national comorbidity survey replication. *Archives of General Psychiatry, 62,* 593–602.

Kiosses, D. N., Teri, L., Velligan, D. I., & Alexopoulos, G. S. (2011). A home-delivered intervention for depressed, cognitively impaired, disabled elders. *International Journal of Geriatric Psychiatry, 26,* 256–262. doi:10.1002/gps.2521

Lenze, E. J., Hickman, S., Hershey, T., Wendleton, L., Ly, K., Dixon, D., . . . Wetherell, J. L. (2014). Mindfulness-based stress reduction for older adults with worry symptoms and co-occurring cognitive dysfunction. *International Journal of Geriatric Psychiatry.* Advance online publication. doi:10.1002/gps.4086

Lenze, E. J., Mulsant, B. H., Mohlman, J., Shear, M., Dew, M., Schulz, R., . . . Reynolds, C. (2005). Generalized anxiety disorder in late life: Lifetime course and comorbidity with major depressive disorder. *The American Journal of Geriatric Psychiatry, 13,* 77–80. doi:10.1097/00019442-200501000-00011

Lenze, E. J., Mulsant, B. H., Shear, M. K., Schulberg, H. C., Dew, M. A., & Begley, A. E. (2000). Comorbid anxiety disorders in depressed elderly patients. *The American Journal of Psychiatry, 157,* 722–728. doi:10.1176/appi.ajp.157.5.722

Lenze, E. J., Rollman, B. L., Shear, M., Dew, M., Pollock, B. G., Ciliberti, C., . . . Reynolds, C. F., III. (2009). Escitalopram for older adults with generalized anxiety disorder. *JAMA, 301,* 295–303. doi:10.1001/jama.2008.977

Letamendi, A. M., Ayers, C. R., Ruberg, J. L., Singley, D. B., Wilson, J., Chavira, D., . . . Wetherell, J. L. (2013). Illness conceptualizations among older rural Mexican-Americans with anxiety and depression. *Journal of Cross-Cultural Gerontology, 28,* 421–433. doi:10.1007/s10823-013-9211-8

Linden, M., Zubraegel, D., Baer, T., Franke, U., & Schlattmann, P. (2005). Efficacy of cognitive behaviour therapy in generalized anxiety disorders. Results of a controlled clinical trial (Berlin CBT-GAD Study). *Psychotherapy and Psychosomatics, 74*, 36–42. doi:10.1159/000082025

Mantella, R. C., Butters, M. A., Dew, M., Mulsant, B. H., Begley, A. E., Tracey, B., . . . Lenze, E. (2007). Cognitive impairment in late-life generalized anxiety disorder. *The American Journal of Geriatric Psychiatry, 15*, 673–679. doi:10.1097/JGP.0b013e31803111f2

Martens, E. J., de Jonge, P., Na, B., Cohen, B. E., Lett, H., & Whooley, M. A. (2010). Scared to death? Generalized anxiety disorder and cardiovascular events in patients with stable coronary heart disease: The Heart and Soul Study. *Archives of General Psychiatry, 67*, 750–758. doi:10.1001/archgenpsychiatry.2010.74

Metge, C., Grymonpre, R., Dahl, M., & Yogendran, M. (2005). Pharmaceutical use among older adults: Using administrative data to examine medication-related issues. *Canadian Journal on Aging, 24*(Suppl. 1), 81–95. doi:10.1353/cja.2005.0052

Meyer, T. J., Miller, M. L., Metzger, R. L., & Borkovec, T. D. (1990). Development and validation of the Penn State Worry Questionnaire. *Behaviour Research and Therapy, 28*, 487–495. doi:10.1016/0005-7967(90)90135-6

Mezhebovsky, I., Magi, K., She, F., Datto, C., & Eriksson, H. (2013). Double-blind, randomized study of extended release quetiapine fumarate (quetiapine XR) monotherapy in older patients with generalized anxiety disorder. *International Journal of Geriatric Psychiatry, 28*, 615–625. doi:10.1002/gps.3867

Mohlman, J. (2013). Executive skills in older adults with GAD: Relations with clinical variables and CBT outcome. *Journal of Anxiety Disorders, 27*, 131–139. doi:10.1016/j.janxdis.2012.12.001

Mohlman, J., Gorenstein, E. E., Kleber, M., de Jesus, M., Gorman, J. M., & Papp, L. A. (2003). Standard and enhanced cognitive-behavior therapy for late-life generalized anxiety disorder: Two pilot investigations. *The American Journal of Geriatric Psychiatry, 11*, 24–32. doi:10.1097/00019442-200301000-00005

Mohlman, J., & Gorman, J. M. (2005). The role of executive functioning in CBT: A pilot study with anxious older adults. *Behaviour Research and Therapy, 43*, 447–465. doi:10.1016/j.brat.2004.03.007

Norton, J., Ancelin, M., Stewart, R., Berr, C., Ritchie, K., & Carriere, I. (2012). Anxiety symptoms and disorder predict activity limitations in the elderly. *Journal of Affective Disorders*. Advance online publication. doi:10.1016/j.jad.2012.04.002.

Norton, P. J., & Price, E. C. (2007). A meta-analytic review of adult cognitive-behavioral treatment outcome across the anxiety disorders. *Journal of Nervous and Mental Disease, 195*, 521–531. doi:10.1097/01.nmd.0000253843.70149.9a

Pachana, N. A., Byrne, G. J., Siddle, H., Koloski, N., Harley, E., & Arnold, E. (2007). Development and validation of the geriatric anxiety inventory. *International Journal of Psychogeriatrics, 19*, 103–114.

Pariente, A., Dartigues, J., Benichou, J., Letenneur, L., Moore, N., & Fourrier-Réglat, A. (2008). Benzodiazepines and injurious falls in community dwelling elders. *Drugs & Aging, 25*, 61–70. doi:10.2165/00002512-200825010-00007

Pietrzak, R. H., Maruff, P., Woodward, M., Fredrickson, J., Fredrickson, A., Krystal, J. H., . . . Darby, D. (2012). Mild worry symptoms predict decline in learning and memory in healthy older adults: A 2-year prospective cohort study. *The American Journal of Geriatric Psychiatry, 20,* 266–275. doi:10.1097/JGP.0b013e3182107e24

Pinquart, M., & Duberstein, P. R. (2007). Treatment of anxiety disorders in older adults: A meta-analytic comparison behavioral and pharmacological interventions. *The American Journal of Geriatric Psychiatry, 15,* 639–651. doi:10.1097/JGP.0b013e31806841c8

Pinquart, M., Duberstein, P. R., & Lyness, J. M. (2006). Treatments for later life depressive conditions: A meta-analytic comparison of pharmacotherapy and psychotherapy. *The American Journal of Psychiatry, 163,* 1493–1501. doi:10.1176/appi.ajp.163.9.1493

Poikolainen, K. (2000). Risk factors for alcohol dependence: A case-control study. *Alcohol and Alcoholism, 35,* 190–196. doi:10.1093/alcalc/35.2.190

Porensky, E. K., Dew, M. A., Karp, J. F., Skidmore, E., Rollman, B. L., Shear, M. K., & Lenze, E. J. (2009). The burden of late-life generalized anxiety disorder: Effects on disability, health-related quality of life, and healthcare utilization. *The American Journal of Geriatric Psychiatry, 17,* 473–482. doi:10.1097/JGP.0b013e31819b87b2

Randolph, C., Tierney, M. C., Mohr, E., & Chase, T. N. (1998). The Repeatable Battery for the Assessment of Neuropsychological Status (RBANS): Preliminary clinical validity. *Journal of Clinical and Experimental Neuropsychology, 20,* 310–319. doi:10.1076/jcen.20.3.310.823.

Rickard, H. C., Scogin, F., & Keith, S. (1994). A one-year follow-up of relaxation training for elders with subjective anxiety. *The Gerontologist, 34,* 121–122. doi:10.1093/geront/34.1.121

Roest, A. M., Martens, E. J., de Jonge, P., & Denollet, J. (2010). Anxiety and risk of incident coronary heart disease: A meta-analysis. *Journal of the American College of Cardiology, 56,* 38–46. doi:10.1016/j.jacc.2010.03.034

Roest, A. M., Zuidersma, M., & de Jonge, P. (2012). Myocardial infarction and generalised anxiety disorder: 10-year follow-up. *The British Journal of Psychiatry, 200,* 324–329. doi:10.1192/bjp.bp.111.103549

Sallis, J. F., Lichstein, K. L., Clarkson, A. D., Stalgaitis, S., & Campbell, M. (1983). Anxiety and depression management for the elderly. *International Journal of Behavioral Geriatrics, 1,* 3–12.

Schaub, R. T., & Linden, M. (2000). Anxiety and anxiety disorders in the old and very old—results from the Berlin Aging Study (BASE). *Comprehensive Psychiatry, 41,* 48–54. doi:10.1016/S0010-440X(00)80008-5

Schultz, S. K., Moser, D. J., Bishop, J. R., & Ellingrod, V. L. (2005). Phobic anxiety in late-life in relationship to cognition and 5HTTLPR polymorphism. *Psychiatric Genetics, 15,* 305–306. doi:10.1097/00041444-200512000-00016

Schuurmans, J., Comijs, H., Emmelkamp, P. M. G., Gundy, C. M. M., Weijnen, I., van den Hout, M., & van Dyck, R. (2006). A randomized, controlled trial of the effectiveness of cognitive-behavioral therapy and sertraline versus a waitlist control group for anxiety disorders in older adults. *The American Journal of Geriatric Psychiatry, 14*, 255–263. doi:10.1097/01.JGP.0000196629.19634.00

Schuurmans, J., Comijs, H., Emmelkamp, P., Weijnen, I., van den Hout, M., & van Dyck, R. (2009). Long-term effectiveness and prediction of treatment outcome in cognitive behavioral therapy and sertraline for late-life anxiety disorders. *International Psychogeriatrics/IPA, 21*, 1148–1159. doi:10.1017/S1041610209990536

Scogin, F., Rickard, H. C., Keith, S., Wilson, J., & McElreath, L. (1992). Progressive and imaginal relaxation training for elderly persons with subjective anxiety. *Psychology and Aging, 7*, 419–424. doi:10.1037/0882-7974.7.3.419

Segal, D. L., June, A., Payne, M., Coolidge, F. L., & Yochim, B. (2010). Development and initial validation of a self-report assessment tool for anxiety among older adults: The Geriatric Anxiety Scale. *Journal of Anxiety Disorders, 24*, 709–714. doi:10.1016/j.janxdis.2010.05.002

Serfaty, M. A., Haworth, D., Blanchard, M., Buszewicz, M., Murad, S., & King, M. (2009). Clinical effectiveness of individual cognitive behavioral therapy for depressed older people in primary care: A randomized controlled trial. *Archives of General Psychiatry, 66*, 1332–1340. doi:10.1001/archgenpsychiatry.2009.165

Smoller, J. W., Pollack, M. H., & Wassertheil-Smoller, S. (2007). Panic attacks and risk of incident cardiovascular events among postmenopausal women in the women's health initiative observational study. *Archives of General Psychiatry, 64*, 1153–1160. doi:10.1001/archpsyc.64.10.1153

Spielberger, C. D., Gorsuch, R. L., Lushene, R., Vagg, P. R., & Jacobs, G. A. (1983). *Manual for the state-trait anxiety inventory*. Palo Alto, CA: Consulting Psychologists Press.

Spitzer, R. L., Kroenke, K., Williams, J. W., & Löwe, B. (2006). A brief measure for assessing generalized anxiety disorder: The GAD-7. *Archives of Internal Medicine, 166*, 1092–1097. doi:10.1001/archinte.166.10.1092

Stanley, M. A., Beck, J. G., & Glassco, J. D. (1996). Treatment of generalized anxiety in older adults: A preliminary comparison of cognitive-behavioral and supportive approaches. *Behavior Therapy, 27*, 565–581. doi:10.1016/S0005-7894(96)80044-X

Stanley, M. A., Beck, J. G., Novy, D. M., Averill, P. M., Swann, A. C., Diefenbach, G. J., & Hopko, D. R. (2003). Cognitive-behavioral treatment of late-life generalized anxiety disorder. *Journal of Consulting and Clinical Psychology, 71*, 309–319. doi:10.1037/0022-006X.71.2.309

Stanley, M. A., Wilson, N. L., Amspoker, A. B., Kraus-Schuman, C., Wagener, P. D., Calleo, J. S., . . . Kunik, M. E. (2014). Lay providers can deliver effective cognitive behavior therapy for older adults with generalized anxiety disorder: A randomized trial. *Depression and Anxiety, 31*, 391–401. doi:10.1002/da.22239

Stanley, M. A., Wilson, N. L., Novy, D. M., Rhoades, H. M., Wagener, P. D., Greisinger, A. J., . . . Kunik, M. E. (2009). Cognitive behavior therapy for generalized anxiety disorder among older adults in primary care: A randomized clinical trial. *JAMA, 301*, 1460–1467. doi:10.1001/jama.2009.458

Thorp, S. R., Ayers, C. R., Nuevo, R., Stoddard, J. A., Sorrell, J. T., & Wetherell, J. L. (2009). Meta-analysis comparing different behavioral treatments for late-life anxiety. *The American Journal of Geriatric Psychiatry, 17*, 105–115. doi:10.1097/JGP.0b013e31818b3f7e

Todaro, J. F., Shen, B. J., Raffa, S. D., Tilkemeier, P. L., & Niaura, R. (2007). Prevalence of anxiety disorders in men and women with established coronary heart disease. *Journal of Cardiopulmonary Rehabilitation and Prevention, 27*, 86–91. doi:10.1097/01.HCR.0000265036.24157.e7

Tolin, D. F., Robison, J. T., Gartamide, S., & Blank, K. (2005). Anxiety disorders in older Puerto Rican primary care patients. *The American Journal of Geriatric Psychiatry, 13*, 150–156. doi:10.1097/00019442-200502000-00009

van Balkom, A. J., Beekman, A. T., De Beurs, E., Deeg, D. H., Van Dyck, R., & Van Tilburg, W. (2000). Comorbidity of the anxiety disorders in a community-based older population in the Netherlands. *Acta Psychiatrica Scandinavica, 101*, 37–45. doi:10.1034/j.1600-0447.2000.101001037.x

van't Veer-Tazelaar, P., van Marwijk, H., van Oppen, P., van Hout, H., van der Horst, H., Cuijpers, P., . . . Beekman, A. (2009). Stepped-care prevention of anxiety and depression in late life: A randomized controlled trial. *Archives of General Psychiatry, 66*, 297–304. doi:10.1001/archgenpsychiatry.2008.555

van't Veer-Tazelaar, P. J., van Marwijk, H. J., van Oppen, P., van der Horst, H. E., Smit, F., Cuijpers, P., & Beekman, A. F. (2011). Prevention of late-life anxiety and depression has sustained effects over 24 months: A pragmatic randomized trial. *The American Journal of Geriatric Psychiatry, 19*, 230–239. doi:10.1097/JGP.0b013e3181faee4d

Vasiliadis, H. M., Dionne, P. A., Preville, M., Gentil, L., Berbiche, D., & Latimer, E. (2012). The excess healthcare costs associated with depression and anxiety in elderly living in the community. *The American Journal of Geriatric Psychiatry*. Advance online publication. doi:10.1097/JGP.0b013e318248ae9e

Vögele, C., & von Leupoldt, A. (2008). Mental disorders in chronic obstructive pulmonary disease. *Respiratory Medicine, 102*, 764–773. doi:10.1016/j.rmed.2007.12.006

Wetherell, J. L., Afari, N., Ayers, C. R., Stoddard, J. A., Ruberg, J., Sorrell, J. T., . . . Patterson, T. L. (2011). Acceptance and commitment therapy for generalized anxiety disorder in older adults: A preliminary report. *Behavior Therapy, 42*, 127–134. doi:10.1016/j.beth.2010.07.002

Wetherell, J. L., Ayers, C. R., Sorrell, J. T., Thorp, S. R., Nuevo, R., Belding, W., . . . Patterson, T. L. (2009). Modular psychotherapy for anxiety in older primary care patients. *The American Journal of Geriatric Psychiatry, 17*, 483–492. doi:10.1097/JGP.0b013e3181a31fb5

Wetherell, J. L., & Gatz, M. (2005). The Beck Anxiety Inventory in older adults with generalized anxiety disorder. *Journal of Psychopathology and Behavioral Assessment, 27,* 17–24. doi:10.1007/s10862-005-3261-3

Wetherell, J. L., Gatz, M., & Craske, M. G. (2003). Treatment of generalized anxiety disorder in older adults. *Journal of Consulting and Clinical Psychology, 71,* 31–40. doi:10.1037/0022-006X.71.1.31

Wetherell, J. L., Petkus, A. J., Thorp, S. R., Stein, M. B., Chavira, D. A., Campbell-Sills, L., . . . Roy-Byrne, P. (2013). Age differences in treatment response to a collaborative care intervention for anxiety disorders. *The British Journal of Psychiatry, 203,* 65–72. doi:10.1192/bjp.bp.112.118547

Wetherell, J. L., Petkus, A. J., White, K. S., Nguyen, H., Kornblith, S., Andreescu, C., . . . Lenze, E. J. (2013). Antidepressant medication augmented with cognitive-behavioral therapy for generalized anxiety disorder in older adults. *The American Journal of Psychiatry, 170,* 782–789. doi:10.1176/appi.ajp.2013.12081104

Wolitzky-Taylor, K. B., Castriotta, N., Lenze, E. J., Stanley, M. A., & Craske, M. G. (2010). Anxiety disorders in older adults: A comprehensive review. *Depression and Anxiety, 27,* 190–211. doi:10.1002/da.20653

Wright, R. M., Roumani, Y. F., Boudreau, R., Newman, A. B., Ruby, C. M., Studenski, S. A., . . . Hanlon, J. T. (2009). Effect of central nervous system medication use on decline in cognition in community-dwelling older adults: Findings from the Health, Aging and Body Composition Study. *Journal of the American Geriatrics Society, 57,* 243–250. doi:10.1111/j.1532-5415.2008.02127.x

Wuthrich, V. M., & Rapee, R. M. (2013). Randomised controlled trial of group cognitive behavioural therapy for comorbid anxiety and depression in older adults. *Behaviour Research and Therapy, 51,* 779–786. doi:10.1016/j.brat.2013.09.002

Yesavage, J. A., Brink, T. L., Rose, T. L., Lum, O., Huang, V., Adey, M., & Leirer, V. O. (1983). Development and validation of a geriatric depression screening scale: a preliminary report. *Journal of Psychiatric Research, 17,* 37–49. doi:10.1177/089198879100400310

Zou, J. B., Dear, B. F., Titov, N., Lorian, C. N., Johnston, L., Spence, J., . . . Sachdev, P. (2012). Brief Internet-delivered cognitive behavioral therapy for anxiety in older adults: A feasibility trial. *Journal of Anxiety Disorders, 26,* 650–655. doi:10.1016/j.janxdis.2012.04.002

Zwart, J. A., Dyb, G., Hagen, K., Ødegård, K. J., Dahl, A. A., Bovim, G., & Stovner, L. J. (2003). Depression and anxiety disorders associated with headache frequency. The Nord-Trøndelag Health Study. *European Journal of Neurology, 10,* 147–152. doi:10.1046/j.1468-1331.2003.00551.x

6

EXPOSURE THERAPY FOR LATE-LIFE TRAUMA

JOAN M. COOK AND STEPHANIE DINNEN

Despite considerable evidence from randomized clinical trials of the efficacy of exposure therapy for posttraumatic stress disorder (PTSD), frontline psychotherapists rarely use this treatment (e.g., Becker, Zayfert & Anderson, 2004; Rosen et al., 2004). This chapter describes the application of prolonged exposure (PE), an evidence-based cognitive behavior therapy (CBT) for older adult trauma survivors with PTSD. It also presents the theoretical background for exposure therapy, as well as cultural, disability, and cognitive impairment factors to consider with older adults. Before presenting this information, though, we summarize the changes to the PTSD diagnosis in the *Diagnostic and Statistical Manual of Mental Disorders* (5th ed.; *DSM–5*; American Psychiatric Association, 2013).

The *Diagnostic and Statistical Manual of Mental Disorders* (4th ed., text rev.; *DSM–IV–TR*; American Psychiatric Association, 2000) provides the following diagnostic criteria for PTSD: *Criterion A* (both A1 and A2 must be met) includes A1, the person witnesses, experiences, or is confronted by an

http://dx.doi.org/10.1037/14524-007
Treatment of Late-Life Depression, Anxiety, Trauma, and Substance Abuse, P. A. Areán (Editor)

event(s) that involved actual or threatened death or serious injury, or threat to the physical integrity of others; and A2, the person's response includes intense fear, helplessness, or horror. *Criterion B* addresses re-experiencing symptoms in at least one or more of the following ways: intrusive recollections (B1), distressing nightmares (B2), flashbacks (B3), physiological distress when exposed to reminders of the trauma (B4), and physiological reactivity when exposed to traumatic reminders (B5). *Criterion C* includes at least three or more of the following avoidance symptoms: avoidance of thoughts feelings or conversations associated with the trauma (C1); avoidance of activities, people, or places associated with the stressor (C2); inability to recall important aspects of the trauma (C3); diminished interest in significant activities (C4); detachment from others (C5); restricted range of affect (C6); and sense of a foreshortened future (C7). *Criterion D* requires at least two or more of the following hyperarousal symptoms: sleep problems (D1), irritability (D2), concentration difficulties (D3), hypervigilance (D4), and exaggerated startle response (D5). *Criterion E*, which requires a duration of at least on 1 month, can be acute (i.e., symptoms last fewer than 3 months); chronic (i.e., symptoms last more than 3 months); or with delayed onset (i.e., symptoms last at least 6 months between the traumatic event and their onset). *Criterion F* represents significant distress or functional impairment.

In the *DSM–5* criteria for PTSD, the definition of a *traumatic event* has changed, and a new cluster of symptoms has been included. Although the *DSM–5* has retained most of the 17 symptoms (with some modifications) that were in the *DSM–IV–TR*, it has added three: pervasive negative emotional state, persistent distorted blame of self or others, and reckless or self-destructive behavior. An important change from the *DSM–IV–TR* is that the *DSM–5* no longer categorizes PTSD within Anxiety Disorders.

Although there has been much debate about the validity of the Criterion A1 construct qualifying traumatic stressors, the *DSM–5* has upheld its utility to the diagnosis of PTSD. Critics of the *DSM–IV–TR* A1 definition found it either too broad (i.e., a loosening of criteria about which events are considered "trauma") or arbitrarily restrictive (i.e., the presence of symptom criteria matters more than the specifics of the event) and that it focused too much on etiological factors while minimizing temporal ones. Criterion A1 remains, with new language that defines *qualifying events* as those involving direct exposure to actual or threatened death and actual or threatened serious injury to self or others. *Indirect exposure* has been limited to a person's learning about the traumatic exposure of a loved one or close friend, or about grievous injury, unnatural death, or serious assault to others and includes work-related exposure to traumatic death and injury (e.g., by emergency personnel following mass tragedies). Importantly, in congruence with the literature, the A1 language now excludes the witnessing of traumatic events via media outlets (e.g., television, Internet, movies). In addition, following the review of substantial and convincing literature that PTSD can develop in the absence of such feelings (Friedman, Resick, Bryant, & Brewin, 2011), *DSM–5* has eliminated the A2 criterion "intense feelings of helplessness, fear or horror."

One of the more important changes in the *DSM–5* PTSD diagnosis is the adoption of a four-factor model of symptom clusters—B, re-experiencing; C, avoidance; D, arousal; and E, dysphoria—in favor of the previous three-factor model—B, re-experiencing; C, avoidance/numbing; and D, hyperarousal—in the *DSM–IV–TR*. Criterion B1 has been limited to spontaneous, intrusive, and distressing memories and now excludes more generalized thoughts or ruminations. Criterion B2 (i.e., traumatic nightmares) no longer requires the dream to reproduce the traumatic event, but instead includes the more broad "trauma-related material." Criterion B3 (i.e., flashbacks) remains the same, although with clearer language that explains flashbacks as a dissociative reaction in which the person feels or acts as if he or she is re-experiencing the trauma. Criteria B4 and B5 remain unchanged. *DSM–IV–TR* Criterion C was divided into *DSM–5* Criterion C (i.e., avoidance) and D (i.e., negative alterations in cognitions or mood) in support of the four-factor model. *DSM–5* Criterion C includes C1 (i.e., avoidance of thoughts, feelings, or conversations associated with the stressor) and C2 (i.e., avoidance of activities, places, or people associated with the stressor). *DSM–5* Criterion D now includes the remaining symptoms (formerly known as C3–C7) of *DSM–5* Criterion C with the addition of two symptoms: pervasive negative emotional state (i.e., horror, shame, guilt, fear) and persistent distorted blame of self or others. *DSM–5* Criterion E became the former *DSM–IV* Criterion D (i.e., insomnia, problems in concentration, hyperarousal, and startle reactions) and included a change from "irritability" in Criterion D2 to "new onset post-traumatic aggressive behavior" and the addition of a symptom supported by emerging literature: reckless or self-destructive behavior. The language of Criterion F, the duration, was modified so that the former label "With Delayed Onset" is now "With Delayed Expression" to reflect that a diagnosis of PTSD in the complete absence of prior symptoms is rare and is more accurately subsyndromal PTSD symptoms that later escalate. In addition, neither partial/subsyndromal PTSD nor complex PTSD (currently classified under Disorders of Extreme Stress, Not Otherwise Specified—DESNOS) was believed to warrant unique diagnostic standing (Friedman et al., 2011).

CASE DESCRIPTION

Mary, a 72-year-old Caucasian, Irish Catholic widow, presented to her primary care physician with difficulties concentrating and sleeping, general nervousness, increased heart palpitations, and sweating. After numerous diagnostic procedures revealed no medical illness, Mary's physician probed into the history of her symptoms. In taking a thorough assessment, the physician learned that Mary lived alone in a high-rise building in Manhattan, New York, below Canal Street and near the former World Trade Center. From her apartment, she had a close view of the former Twin Towers and reported that one of her greatest daily pleasures was watching the comings and goings of passersby.

On September 11, 2001, Mary diverged from her usual midmorning routine of going to a local senior center; instead, she remained home to perform housecleaning tasks. When the first plane hit one of the towers, Mary reported hearing a "deafening" noise and felt the "ground shake." From her window, she witnessed the first tower burning. Mary described feeling mesmerized like she was "in a trance," and she couldn't take her eyes off the building. She watched in horror and disbelief as a second plane hit the other tower, victims jumped from high windows to their death, and both towers collapsed. She heard sirens and people screaming. Shortly thereafter, an intensely dense, dark dust cloud obscured her view. Mary had little recollection of what happened subsequently.

Mary typically wore hearing aids, but she did not wear them the morning of September 11. Neighbors or the superintendent may have knocked on her door to help her evacuate the apartment building. However, if they did so, she did not hear them. Mary's only daughter had moved to South Florida the year before, and Mary had no immediate family members or other capable support people nearby. Between the breakdown of communications (telephone and wireless lines were interrupted) and the inability of anyone to gain access to the "frozen zone," the blockaded area near the terroristic attacks, Mary remained in her apartment for 3 days before being "rescued."

During that time, power outages caused television, telephone, radio, and Internet service interruptions, and newspapers and mail were not delivered. Without electricity, the apartment building had no lights, no refrigeration for fresh food, and no working elevators. Mary's building manager called a meeting in the lobby for residents who had not evacuated and explained what had happened. Mary did not wear her hearing aids and felt confused by the information. He instructed residents to stay in their apartments for their safety until rescue workers removed them. While she waited, Mary could hear sirens and F-16 aircraft. She thought another attack was occurring and felt helpless, thinking she might die alone. Because travel was restricted—bridges and tunnels in and out of Manhattan were closed for security reasons—and telephone communication was unreliable, her daughter was unable to contact Mary until 2 days after the attacks. For the next several months, Mary spent a lot of time watching media coverage of the terroristic attacks on the television.

During the year following the attacks, many changes occurred for Mary. Numerous people moved out of the apartment building. Several of Mary's older neighbors either moved to join family members out of town or moved to semi-independent living facilities in other New York boroughs. Mary had lived in this particular apartment her entire adult life, had raised her daughter there, and was reticent to leave, although her daughter offered that Mary could move to Florida and live near her. Mary only minimally attended church and discontinued her participation at the local senior center.

Changes also occurred in the community. Local businesses and stores that Mary frequented (e.g., dry cleaners, delicatessen) went out of business and the neighborhood had a heightened police presence, thus greatly disrupting her immediate surroundings and daily routine. In addition, a foul odor from the explosions and collapse filled the air, so Mary increasingly kept her apartment windows closed. She felt like she was losing contact with the outside world.

EXPOSURE THERAPY: THEORETICAL BACKGROUND AND APPLICATION TO AGING

CBT has been found to be the most efficacious treatment approach for PTSD (Foa, Keane, Friedman, & Cohen, 2009). The most commonly studied therapy under the umbrella of CBT across trauma populations is *exposure therapy* (for a review, see Cahill, Rothbaum, Resick, & Follette, 2009), treatment that includes a form of imaginal or in vivo exposure to traumatic memories and situations avoided because of the traumatic reminders. Of the class of treatments under exposure therapy, PE (Foa, Hembree, & Rothbaum, 2007) is the most widely studied and is well validated (Cahill et al., 2009). In a review of 13 randomized controlled trials of PE with adolescents and adults, this intervention was found to be highly effective in treating PTSD and significantly more effective than inactive (i.e., waiting list) and active (i.e., psychological placebo) control conditions (Powers, Halpern, Ferenschak, Gillihan, & Foa, 2010).

PE is based on the theory of *emotional processing* (Foa & Kozak, 1986), which posits that fear is a structure represented in the memory by three features: (a) feared stimuli (e.g., riding in a car); (b) fear-based physiological responses (e.g., quickened breath); and (c) construal of meaning about the stimuli and response (e.g., "We're going to crash"). It is believed that PTSD results when an individual generalizes fears to all stimuli and responses, thus creating a view of the world as constantly dangerous and of the person as helpless or incompetent in it. When a person inaccurately perceives either stimuli as dangerous or the meaning construed from stimuli or response as threatening, the result can be a pathological, overly intense response that can interfere with daily functioning.

PE is typically delivered in eight to 15 weekly or biweekly 90-minute sessions. It consists of four main components: (a) psychoeducation, (b) breathing retraining, (c) imaginal exposure, and (d) in vivo exposure (Foa et al., 2007). *Psychoeducation* includes the treatment rationale, general information about PTSD, an explanation of common reactions to trauma, and discussion about a singular index trauma judged to be the most upsetting. *Breathing retraining* is taught as a means of reducing anxiety to allow for engagement in necessary therapeutic tasks. *Imaginal exposure* involves the client's repeated recounting aloud of details of the most disturbing traumatic event. Typically, with eyes closed for 30 to 60 minutes, the client details descriptions of the event, as well as related thoughts and feelings, using present tense. *In vivo exposure* is used between therapy sessions as a means of bringing the client into contact with situations, places, or objects he or she has avoided following a trauma.

Some have debated the appropriateness of exposure therapy in traumatized older adults (Coleman, 1999; Hyer & Woods, 1998; Kruse & Schmitt, 1999). One argument against using exposure with this population is the potential for increased physiological arousal and decreased cognitive performance—in particular, a belief that this possibility can be harmful and unproductive in older adults who may have comorbid physical or cognitive ailments (Hyer & Woods, 1998).

Physiological arousal, however, is considered a marker of emotional engagement with the trauma memory, and thus is thought to be a required component of successful exposure therapy (Jaycox, Foa, & Morral, 1998). Supporters of exposure therapies in older adults agree that physiological arousal is an expected but tolerable component in aging clients (Thorp, Sones, & Cook, 2011). In the absence of empirical data, it seems reasonable to proceed with appropriate caution and monitor clients at great risk from high arousal, such as those with serious cardiac or respiratory problems (Cook, Schnurr & Foa, 2004). One suggestion for managing potential complications resulting from increased physiological arousal is to remain in consultation with the older adult's primary physician and to monitor arousal levels by asking the client if the experience is physically uncomfortable and to what degree (Thorp et al., 2011).

Case studies of older adult clients using elements of exposure therapy (i.e., imaginal exposure only, in vivo exposure only, and one pilot study using a full, manualized version) support its use in effectively ameliorating symptoms related to trauma and maladaptive posttraumatic response (Cornelius & Kenyon-Jump, 2007; Gamito et al., 2010; Russo, Hersen, Van Hasselt, 2001; Thorp, Stein, Jeste, Patterson, & Wetherell, 2012; Thyer, 1981; Yoder,

Tuerk & Acierno, 2010). Thyer (1981) presented a case study of a 70-year-old woman with phobic disorder who underwent in vivo exposure treatment for a severe fear of dogs following an unprovoked attack. Apparently, after 3 years of supportive psychotherapy, the woman experienced little symptom reduction and further severe functional limitations (e.g., she was unable to leave her home for fear of encountering dogs). After five sessions of in vivo exposure, the woman was acclimated to dogs in the presence of her therapist (e.g., bringing a leashed dog into the room, visits to the humane society, walks past a dog park). She reportedly tolerated well the anxiety induced during exposure sessions. Reduction in symptoms and increase in functioning were achieved and maintained at 6-month follow-up.

In a case study of a 57-year-old woman with PTSD resulting from childhood sexual abuse, Russo, Hersen, and Van Hasselt (2001) successfully applied a range of treatments, such as exposure therapy, to treated PTSD symptomatology. The treatment occurred over 2 years and included supportive psychotherapy, imaginal exposure, and skill generalization. That work suggests that exposure can be successfully applied to recurring PTSD with an older adult.

Cornelius and Kenyon-Jump (2007) applied a 15-session, brief, gradual, exposure-based protocol over 7 months to a 72-year-old African American former police officer who had PTSD from witnessing fatal or near-fatal on-the-job traumatic events. Although this treatment involved both imaginal and in vivo exposure, during the initial sessions brief exposures were conducted and then alternated with relaxation exercises. The authors' stated rationale for not primarily or solely using PE was that they needed to build clinical rapport and that gradual exposure would allow the client to acclimate better to treatment.

Yoder, Tuerk, and Acierno (2010) provided a case study of the application of PE with an 87-year-old World War II veteran and former prisoner of war presenting with moderate PTSD and mild depression. Treatment included seven PE sessions. Although the client was diagnosed with atrial fibrillation, a common cardiac arrhythmia, routine monitoring by his cardiologist indicated no adverse physiological changes during the course of treatment. By the conclusion of the seventh session, the client no longer met criteria for PTSD or depression.

In a small randomized controlled trial involving 10 older war veterans in Portugal, Gamito and colleagues (2010) compared virtual reality exposure therapy (involving computer graphics, body tracking devices, and visual and other sensory input to immerse clients in a computer-generated virtual environment); imaginal exposure; and wait-list control. The two active treatment conditions consisted of 12 sessions and produced significant changes in depression and anxiety.

The feasibility and preliminary efficacy of PE were assessed in 14 older male U.S. veterans with PTSD (Thorp et al., 2012). The clients ranged in age from 56 to 78, with a mean of 63; most were Caucasian. Although almost half of the clients reported that combat was their worst traumatic experience, others reported sexual assaults or serious accidents. Therapy consisted of 12 individual, twice weekly, 90-minute sessions. The relatively moderate dropout rate (27%) is consistent with other PTSD psychotherapy studies (for a review, see Hembree, Foa, Dorfan, Street, Kowalski, & Tu, 2003). Of the 11 older veterans who completed this open pilot trial, clinician and self-report measures indicated a significant decrease in PTSD from the extreme to the moderate range in symptoms. Only one of the veterans continued to meet diagnostic criteria for PTSD posttreatment. Those veterans who were prescribed medication showed a more significant decrease in severity than those who were not taking psychotropic medication.

One randomized clinical trial on the treatment of PTSD investigated the role of age on clinical outcomes. In a study of 145 sexual assault survivors with PTSD, older women in PE and younger women in cognitive processing therapy (Resick, & Schnicke, 1993) had the best outcomes (Rizvi, Vogt, & Resick, 2009). The authors suggested that the outcome may have been the result of challenges in changing chronic maladaptive cognitions in older individuals. However, the mean age of the sample was 32, and the authors did not provide an age range. It is likely that this sample did not include many women older than age 65. Clearly, more methodologically rigorous treatment trials are needed involving a range of older trauma survivors with PTSD.

EXPOSURE THERAPY: A CASE ILLUSTRATION

Three years after the September 11th terrorist attacks, Mary's primary care physician referred her to an academic mental health clinic specializing in state-of-the-art treatment for trauma-related psychiatric problems. Mary received a thorough diagnostic assessment that included the administration of the Clinician-Administered PTSD Scale (CAPS; Blake et al., 1995). The CAPS is a 30-item, widely used, gold standard structured interview that measures the frequency on a scale ranging from 0 (*none of the time*) to 4 (*most or all of the time*) and intensity on a scale ranging from 0 (*none*) to 4 (*extreme*) of each *DSM–IV* PTSD symptom. In addition to assessing the 17 PTSD symptoms are numerous other items, including those that assess the effect of symptoms on social and occupational functioning and five associated symptoms (i.e., guilt over acts, survivor guilt, gaps in awareness, depersonalization, derealization).

The most frequently used scoring is referred to as the "1/2 rule," which stipulates that, to count a symptom as present, it must have a frequency of 1 or more and an intensity of 2 or more. A diagnosis of PTSD is given if the person has at least one Criterion B (i.e., re-experiencing) symptom, three Criterion C (i.e., avoidance/numbing) symptoms, and two Criterion D (i.e., hyperarousal) symptoms—in addition to meeting the other diagnostic criteria. Severity scores are typically derived from adding the frequency and intensity ratings for each symptom. For alternative scoring suggestions, see Weathers, Keane, and Davidson (2001).

Although the CAPS has sound psychometric properties for use in adults across a variety of clinical populations and research settings (Weathers et al., 2001), reports of its use in older adults are limited (for a review, see van Zelst & Beekman, 2012). One exception was an investigation in older combat veterans (Hyer, Summers, Boyd, Litaker, & Boudewyns, 1996). In that study, the CAPS was deemed appropriate for diagnosis of PTSD with high internal consistency (a = .95), and using an overall CAPS score of 45 or higher had high specificity, sensitivity, and positive and negative predictive power (Hyer et al., 1996). See the U.S. Department of Veterans Affairs (VA) National Center for PTSD website at http://www.ptsd.va.gov/professional/assessment/adult-int/caps.asp for information on how to obtain a copy of the CAPS and for training on how to administer CAPS.

After administration of the CAPS, Mary was diagnosed with PTSD and major depression. In particular, she reported moderate to severe symptoms in each of the three PTSD symptom clusters (i.e., re-experiencing, hyperarousal, and avoidance). Mary's re-experiencing symptoms included regular nightmares of burning bodies falling from buildings, intrusive memories of the planes striking the towers and the collapse of the buildings, and being distressed when confronted with trauma reminders. Her avoidance symptoms including avoiding thoughts of September 11th and subsequent few days and avoiding situations in which she perceived herself as being most vulnerable (e.g., large crowded areas in New York City, darkness). Her hyperarousal symptoms included difficulty falling and staying asleep, having an exaggerated startle response, and feeling irritable and jumpy.

Having viewed the destruction of the World Trade Center and extremely fearful that New York City would be the target of another terroristic attack, Mary severely limited her activities and refused to use any public transit, such as subway or bus, which had previously been her only means of travel other than walking. In addition, she was no longer able to engage in air travel to visit her daughter and grandchildren in South Florida. Mary was a proud woman who attempted to hide or minimize her distress to others, including her daughter and health care providers.

Mary did not report any prior treatment for psychiatric problems and denied any family history of mental illness. She also denied a current or past history of suicidal ideation or intent. In addition to her present psychiatric symptoms, Mary was filled with intense sadness over the loss of the Twin Towers and the attacks on her beloved city, in which she had lived her entire adult life.

Although Mary denied a history of any other significant traumas, she described a stressful experience that caused her emotional and physical distress. In 1995, a major power outage left New York City and much of the surrounding region without power. While attempting to vacate the city with her daughter, Mary was caught in the crowds, tripped on the sidewalk, and fell. She injured her left leg and required a cane to walk. Occasionally, if covering longer distances, Mary used a wheelchair for comfort and greater mobility. Following a brief stay in an assisted recovery facility, Mary returned to her apartment; a part time home-health aide visited twice weekly for 3 months. Since the experience, Mary has had an increased fear of falling and thus has curtailed several activities she previously enjoyed outside of her apartment.

During her first session, Mary's therapist explained the long and successful tradition of using exposure therapy for anxiety disorders and that PE had been used effectively with a range of trauma survivors. The therapist then presented an overview of and treatment rationale for PE. She explained that the two main procedures used to decrease PTSD symptoms were imaginal and in vivo exposure. After describing these aspects of treatment in full detail, the therapist explained that, in therapy, Mary would confront her distressing memories and reminders to facilitate the processing of the trauma and that, over time, would learn that these memories and reminders are not dangerous and that her anxiety or distress would decrease after repeated and prolonged confrontation. Mary's therapist then taught her a breathing retraining technique to help her learn how to breathe slowly and thus relax. Part of Mary's homework was to read a rationale for treatment handout that was presented in a large print font to facilitate an easier read.

The PTSD Checklist–Civilian version (PCL–C; Weathers, Litz, Herman, Huska, & Keane, 1993) was used weekly throughout treatment to monitor PTSD symptoms. The PTSD Checklist (PCL) is a 17-item, self-report measure of the 17 *DSM–IV* symptoms of PTSD. Symptoms are rated on a 5-point Likert scale ranging from 1 (*not at all*) to 5 (*extremely*) as the extent to which they bothered the client in the previous month, and the PCL yields a summed total score (range is 17–85). The PCL is a reliable measure for use with community-dwelling and older primary care patients who have been exposed to trauma (Cook, Elhai, & Areán, 2005). Receiver operating characteristic analyses revealed that a PCL score of 37 achieved optimal sensitivity and specificity when compared to the PCL's algorithm-derived PTSD diagnosis (Cook et al., 2005). In addition, in each session, Mary's progress with homework was reviewed.

During the second session, Mary learned about common reactions to trauma and was surprised those symptoms had a name; she had previously assumed she was "going crazy." In addition, her therapist shared findings from recent research, namely, a national web-based survey conducted 1 to 2 months after the September 11th attacks (Schlenger et al., 2002). The findings indicated that among females in New York City, being at the World Trade Center and media exposure were related to PTSD. Mary responded, "So it's not just me?" After the therapist normalized and validated Mary's reactions to September 11th, she showed a videotape of the *Dateline NBC* program in which a rape survivor talked about her experiences with PE. Mary explained that she was afraid to face her fears and thought her symptoms might get worse. She was concerned about the "intensity" of the treatment. She questioned the rationale for deliberately thinking about September 11th and the days after the attacks and engaging in feared activities. She was afraid she would be unable to tolerate facing the memories and reminders and might start crying and never stop. After the therapist reiterated the rationale for exposure treatment, Mary reported that she believed that completing the therapy would boost her confidence.

Mary's therapist provided basic psychoeducation that exposure, although uncomfortable at first, is effective in that it helps to: (a) discriminate true from perceived threats, (b) habituate to safe stimuli over time, (c) show that emotional distress will not last forever, and (d) gain mastery over previously avoided situations and memories. The therapist told Mary that it is normal to feel uncomfortable doing previously avoided activities or remembering the events of September 11th.

Mary and her therapist then constructed an in vivo hierarchy of avoided stimuli and situations. The list was long and included objects or situations directly related to her September 11th trauma and those that now evoked anxiety through the generalization of fear: hearing fire trucks or ambulances; media reminders of Homeland Security alerts; visiting the former World Trade Center site; being in crowded places (e.g., Times Square, Grand Central Station); watching news on the Iraq War; seeing groups of cops, national guard, or barricades; seeing airplanes or jets in patrolling the skies; and taking public transit. The therapist introduced the Subjective Units of Distress Scale (Wolpe, 1969) and explained that it would serve as an emotional thermometer to how well Mary was doing through the imaginal exposure portion of the sessions and during her in vivo homework assignments. They worked collaboratively to assign a Subjective Units of Distress Scale rating as to how much each experience on the list would elicit distress or discomfort in Mary if she were to engage in it right now. Afterward, the therapist discussed how

Mary would systematically and gradually approach these feared but otherwise safe objects and situations with the goals of reducing her fear.

In addition, Mary and her therapist made a list of pleasurable activities that she used to enjoy but no longer engaged in after September 11th, such as attending community center functions, visiting Central Park, and taking the bus with her friend to church. She was encouraged to begin to engage in some of these activities, starting with easier tasks. Over the next week, Mary was asked to review the in vivo list of avoided situations to see if she needed to add any other items to the list and to practice two in vivo exposures and attend one pleasant event.

The next week, Mary was late arriving at the third session. She reported that she was extremely anxious and had thought about skipping the session. Mary completed her first imaginal exposure for 45 minutes without interruption. She was instructed to close her eyes and describe her experiences on September 11th in the present tense with as much sensory information as she could remember. In the session, Mary was extremely nervous. She cried throughout the imaginal exposure and subsequently reported that she felt physically and psychologically weak. The therapist praised Mary for attending the session and for her bravery in facing her traumatic memories.

In the fourth session, Mary said that she was again reluctant to engage in imaginal exposure. As a result, she recounted her story in a monotone voice, with a flat affect as opposed to "reliving" the experience. Still, the therapist praised Mary for attending session and for her courage in facing her memories.

Over the next 6 weeks, Mary continued to participate in imaginal exposure during sessions. Her therapist gently reminded her to engage in the trauma memory by keeping her eyes closed, telling her experiences in the present tense, and recalling as many sensory details as possible. Mary actively listened to audiotapes of each session at least one time over the previous week and to the audiotape of her imaginal exposure at least once a day. She continued to practice her in vivo exposure homework, sometimes with the help of a close friend from church.

At the conclusion of treatment, Mary no longer met full criteria for PTSD. She reported that her memory of that fateful day was now clearer and less distressing. She said that she had gained new perceptions of her strengths and how well she had coped and survived those 3 days while she waited to be evacuated. In addition, now that she was feeling better, Mary was able to acknowledge that she had successfully coped with numerous past challenges throughout her life.

Mary also was validated in her belief that the threat of terrorist attacks is a reality and New York City may be a high-target area. Her therapist introduced the concept of relative risk appraisal (Marshall et al., 2007) to help

Mary understand how her previous experiences (i.e., power outage in 1995 and September 11th) and expectations (i.e., New York City is inherently dangerous) derived from those experiences were influencing her perception of current and future events. With her therapist's help, Mary was able to acknowledge that some risk is involved in everyday activities but that the risk of adverse outcomes is relatively low compared with the necessity of those activities to ongoing functioning. Mary was able to see the difference between the general risk of another potential terrorist attack on the United States and the risk of her being in the exact city, on the exact subway car, at the exact time of a potential attack. Furthermore, the therapist asked Mary to list the benefits and losses, such as air, subway, or bus travel, associated with avoiding reminders of September 11th. For Mary, the loss she felt most by refusing to take any public transit was the growing disconnect between herself and her daughter and grandchildren, whom Mary had stopped visiting. Mary's therapist asked her to decide if she felt the consequence of her negative risk appraisal of any public transportation was worth the loss of her visits to her family in Florida. While acknowledging that Mary's assessment of New York City as at risk for an attack, the therapist worked with Mary to successfully adapt to the likelihood of ongoing threat.

Mary received reassurances from her therapist that lessons learned from September 11th involved major governmental review and policy changes on how to create a communications system to reach vulnerable populations, such as older and homebound adults, and that New York City was now better prepared for emergency planning (Renne, Sanchez, & Litman, 2008). Mary's therapist helped her identify the nearest emergency evacuation "pickup point" to her apartment, a service offered by the city's Office of Emergency Management for carless residents when mass evacuations are ordered. Furthermore, Mary's therapist printed out instructions for residents seeking public shelter—23 reception centers across the city would transport residents to shelters around the city's many boroughs—and helped Mary locate the nearest shelter. Because of Mary's walking limitations, the therapist encouraged Mary to place a phone call to the local Red Cross, which noted that, should it be necessary, Mary would require transportation to a reception center.

To help Mary gain a sense of control and prepare for all types of potential disasters in the future, her therapist worked with her to create an emergency box and a "go-bag." The emergency box included important documents, an extra set of apartment keys, a first-aid kit, a battery-operated radio, a flashlight, a blanket, a week's supply of medication, nonperishable food, water, and cash. The go-bag included a list of important phone numbers of family members, doctors, and pharmacies, plus Mary's prescriptions. That strategy enabled Mary to feel more in control and less anxious about the potential for attacks.

The therapist invited Mary to call if she ever needed a "tune-up" of the skills she had learned. She reminded Mary that anniversary reactions are normal and typically resolve on their own.

CULTURE, DISABILITY, AND COGNITIVE IMPAIRMENT CONSIDERATIONS

Relatively little is known about how the issues of culture, disability, and cognitive impairment influence the lives of older adult trauma survivors. For example, limited information exists about the rates of traumatic exposure and the experience and expression of mental health effects in older adults from various cultures (e.g., ethnicities or races), disabilities, and levels of cognitive functioning. Moreover, scant attention has been paid to how these factors influence the assessment and treatment of trauma-related distress, particularly PTSD, in older populations.

Culture

Culture has been ascribed varied definitions and can encompass a person or group's implicit and explicit knowledge, experience, beliefs, values, attitudes, meanings, hierarchies, or religion, among other factors (Brown, 2008). Race and ethnicity, although typically associated with cultural diversity, are thus only two forms of diversity.

To date, research on how ethnicity influences the rates of trauma and PTSD in older adults has focused primarily on differences between non-Hispanic Caucasians and African Americans and Caribbean Blacks. For example, the risk of developing PTSD decreased after young adulthood for non-Hispanic Caucasians but continued throughout the adult lifespan for African Americans and Caribbean Blacks (Himle, Baser, Taylor, Campbell, & Jackson, 2009). In large community samples, older African Americans and Caribbean Blacks had a higher risk for PTSD than older Caucasians. Increased vulnerability for PTSD in these two groups may be the result of higher exposure to trauma and race-related oppression and stressors. Data from a convenience sample using self-report indicated a different clinical picture. In community-residing Caucasian and African American older adult victims of recent crime, no differences existed in the prevalence of overall PTSD or its three symptom clusters (Mainous, Smith, Acierno, & Geesey, 2005). However, among those with a nonphysical trauma, Caucasians were more likely to exceed the PTSD diagnostic threshold for hyperarousal symptoms. Mainous and colleagues (2005) suggested that, because of long-standing cultural experiences, African Americans may have had to develop different coping strategies and thus respond to objectively less dangerous situations with less fear-related arousal.

Much of the early work on ethnocultural aspects of trauma and PTSD used a Western point of view and has been criticized as ethnocentric or biased. Over the past 2 decades, understanding of indigenous expressions of distress, sensitivity in assessment, and language has increased (Marsella, Friedman, & Spain, 1992).

The limited information on the experience of trauma and its treatment in cross-culturally diverse older adults comes primarily from refugee or immigrant populations (e.g., Chung, 2003; Lew, 1991; Strug & Mason, 2007). For example, Lew (1991) proposed interventions for improving the use of mental health services among older adult refugees, many of whom have high rates of traumatic exposure. In addition, refugees typically experience a cadre of stressors: social (e.g., little mental health education), economic (e.g., limited access to transportation), and cultural (e.g., high stigmas against emotional expression). Interventions suggested to address these barriers include community outreach, the use of cultural and linguistic intermediaries between older refugees and Western providers, and the implementation of psychoeducational classes in convenient locations (e.g., religious or cultural centers).

In a qualitative investigation of the effect of September 11th on older Chinese and Hispanic immigrants in New York City, Strug and Mason (2007) found that cultural values were associated with coping strategies. For instance, with relatively poor English language skills and a strong belief in destiny, many older Hispanic people reported that, to cope, they engaged in church attendance and private prayer. In addition, many older Hispanic individuals also had low socioeconomic status, poor health, and eroding social supports that limited their ability to cope effectively. Similarly, many older immigrants from Chinatown did not engage in communication of their private matters and feelings; instead, they engaged in activities to distract themselves from thinking about September 11th (Chung, 2003). Despite intense feelings of anxiety and sadness, those groups did not seek counseling from formal traditional mental health agencies, because they may have viewed such services with mistrust. Thus, it may be necessary to devise or seek alternative models. Chung (2003) suggested service recommendations for older minority trauma survivors, namely, that services be provided by indigenous groups that function both as a surrogate support network and a promoter of self-help. She also advocated for the use of storytelling in group settings to promote social interaction and bonding.

Given the vast differences across and within ethnoracial and cultural groups, it may be impossible to create concrete and singular adaptations to treatments to fit differing older minority populations. Instead, culturally competent practice begins a collaborative discussion between therapist and client about the client's ethnocultural and individual expectations, goals, and preferences (Brown, 2008).

Treatment expectations likely differ within cultures and influence engagement in therapy. A culturally sensitive and supportive therapist would likely assist in the recovery process. However, although it is important to understand how many variables may influence the experience and expression of trauma-related distress, it is also essential to not stereotype people because of their ethnicity, culture, age, or disability status in regard to how well they are functioning posttrauma or how well they will respond to psychological intervention.

Marshall and Suh (2003) discussed the influence of ethnicity and culture on CBT dropout and outcome for adult trauma survivors. Although exposure therapies have been identified as first-line treatment for adults with PTSD, some researchers have questioned its application to non-Western populations (Asukai, Saito, Tsuruta, Kishimoto, & Nishikawa, 2010). However, several studies have reported on the successful application of CBT in culturally or ethnically diverse immigrant and refugee populations (Asukai et al., 2010; Otto & Hinton, 2006; Otto et al., 2003; Paunovic & Ost, 2001). Yet, little of that research has focused on ethnocultural considerations of PTSD in older populations.

Paunovic and Ost (2001) reported on a randomized controlled trial comparing the efficacy of CBT and exposure therapy in a group of refugees seeking asylum in Sweden. Participants were aged 18 to 60 years, and no information was provided on refugee ethnicity. Comparable reductions in PTSD and symptoms of anxiety and depression were found between the two treatments, and, in both treatment gains, were maintained at 6-month follow-up. However, study selection criteria included the ability to speak Swedish fluently (thus negating any language challenges), and a maximum age of 60 years limited generalizations to older refugee populations.

In a randomized controlled trial, Asukai and colleagues (2010) compared PE with treatment as usual in Japanese civilians. They conducted the study without the use of cultural modifications to evaluate the efficacy of PE as true to its original format in non-Western populations. The 24 participants were predominately female, with crime- or accident-related PTSD. Findings revealed greater reductions in PTSD and depressive symptoms and general psychopathology in the PE group compared with the comparison condition. Furthermore, dropout rates (i.e., about 20%) for the PE group were no higher than those reported in Western-based treatment research. Again, because the authors did not report participants' age range, it is unclear how those results would generalize to non-Western or culturally diverse older adults.

Otto and Hinton (2006) described an innovative, detailed guide for modifying exposure-based CBT for severely traumatized Cambodian refugees with PTSD. That work included overcoming numerous challenges; for example, the refugees spoke little to no English and were nonliterate in both languages and, because of clinical resources, treatment was offered in a group format and adapted to focus on somatic presentations and cultural interpretations of the symptoms. Thus, for these and several other reasons, the providers did not use imaginal and in vivo exposure. Rather, with the help of interpreters, they taught about the process of exposure and helped the clients engage in *interoceptive exposure*, a technique that helps clients directly confront feared bodily sensations in a controlled, safe manner typically through hyperventilation, exercise, or holding of one's breath. The decision to not directly process the trauma but, rather, help clients to learn to change the meaning of trauma cues so that intense emotions were not elicited, proved successful. To convey the core concepts of treatment, the providers used metaphors and culturally relevant examples (e.g., compared the focus on skills acquisition to the learning of steps in making a noodle dish, used a lotus blossom as the relaxation imagery). The pilot investigation indicated large effect sizes for CBT on measures of fears of somatic sensations (Otto et al., 2003).

Some cultures may consider the repeated questioning required in PE and the larger umbrella of CBT to be offensive or intrusive. For instance, in traditional Asian cultures, emotion moderation is a virtue, and repetitively discussing emotional experiences in detail is viewed as inappropriate (Chu, Huynh, & Areán, 2012). Conversely, some cultures, such as certain American Indian tribes, value narrative storytelling and may respond well to the cohesive narrative that PE helps people develop (Mays et al., 2009). To foster alliance in working with a minority client, a therapist, particularly one of a dominant majority culture, should highlight the collaborative nature of the therapeutic relationship. Although some client values may be at odds with Western thoughts and beliefs, it is important to not question the rationality or validity of culturally based views, but, rather, to focus on their utility in a given situation. The therapist needs to respect culturally based preferences for individual or group therapy whenever possible. It is likewise important to acknowledge the helpfulness of culturally based strengths within the person and community (Brown, 2008).

Disability

Disability can be defined as changes or challenges to the body or mind's functional ability in a way that interferes with one or more life functions (Brown, 2008). Disability can be a social, developmental, or acquired construct. For instance, a person may be born with a disability (i.e., developed in utero) or may acquire a disability later in life through an accident, such as traumatic brain injury. However, not all functional limitations are disabling to all people (e.g., mild to moderate problems with hearing may be circumvented by the use of hearing aids). Having a disability is believed to greatly increase the risk of traumatic exposure (Brown, 2008). Subsequently, some disabilities may result from the trauma itself (e.g., combat-induced blast injury).

People with disabilities are part of a minority culture; thus, it is important to pay careful attention to potential *ableism*—bias against people with disabilities—when considering assessment, diagnosis, and treatment (Brown, 2008; Hays, 2009; Olkin, 1999). For instance, a therapist should not assume that a disability is itself traumatizing or stressful. Like being part of a racial, sexual orientation, or gender minority, having a disability can complicate traumatic experiences and posttraumatic reactions. Engaging in culturally competent practice includes assessing and being aware of physical and cognitive barriers to caring for people with disabilities (e.g., becoming a Medicare approved provider, accommodation of service animals; Brown, 2008). Older adults may experience age-related disabilities, such as hearing loss, mobility issues, or vision impairment that require treatment modifications, including reliance on public or senior-service transportation, use of large print handouts, or greater reliance on imaginal exposure exercises when an adult cannot physically do in vivo exposure.

Cognitive Impairments

Studies of PTSD or psychiatric distress in physically and mentally impaired older disaster survivors are almost nonexistent, thus highlighting an important gap in the literature (for a review, see Cook & Elmore, 2009). The one exception involved a longitudinal data collection in older adults in the New York area, pre- and post-September 11th, who had applied for vision rehabilitation (Brennan, Horowitz, & Reinhardt, 2003). Although depression spiked in the 4 days immediately following September 11th, no significant differences existed in depression before or after the terroristic attacks.

Cognitive impairment is defined along a continuum of severity. *Mild cognitive impairment* involves deficits in memory that do not significantly affect day-to-day functional abilities (Sachs et al., 2011). *Mild to moderate cognitive impairment* may interfere with attention, language, memory, judgment, reading, and writing. When cognitive impairment is severe enough to affect daily functioning, it is typically classified as *dementia*.

Until recently, aged individuals with cognitive impairments have been largely excluded from studies of PTSD; thus, comparatively little is known about trauma and PTSD and their relationship to cognitive impairments of later life. Some evidence suggests that exposure to extreme trauma (e.g., concentration camp survivors, captivity) can lead to neurological concomitants years after the trauma (Golier et al., 2002; Sutker, Vasterling, Brailey, & Allain, 1995). For example, former prisoners of war with severe trauma-induced weight loss often have long-term deficits in cognitive abilities compared with former prisoners of war with lower weight loss percentages and combat veterans who were not prisoners of war (Sutker et al., 1995).

One study that examined a sample of women age 40 years or older (having an average age of 76) with probable Alzheimer's disease found that 17.5% of participants reported spousal abuse with head trauma on five or more occasions and lost consciousness on two or more occasions (Leung, Thompson, & Weaver, 2006). The likelihood of cognitive impairments in women who had experienced repeated instances of spousal abuse with head trauma were nearly four times as high as in women who had not experienced that type of abuse. These women reported that the majority of the abuse had occurred more than 30 years earlier.

Two recent empirical investigations have presented the strongest evidence to date of a connection between PTSD and cognitive impairment (Qureshi et al., 2010; Yaffe et al., 2010). Yaffe and colleagues (2010) followed more than 181,000 military veterans over a 6-year period, including more than 53,000 with PTSD. Those with PTSD were more than twice as likely to develop dementia. In another study, older veterans with PTSD or who had received a Purple Heart were compared to age- and gender-matched veterans with no PTSD or Purple Heart (Qureshi et al., 2010). A greater prevalence and incidence of dementia was found in older veterans with PTSD. Those with PTSD but who were not Purple Heart recipients had almost twice the odds of developing dementia compared to those who did not have PTSD but had received a Purple Heart or compared to the comparison groups.

Explanations for why severe and prolonged exposure to trauma or PTSD may put an aged individual at higher risk for cognitive deficits and dementia vary. One has posited that trauma is the cause of both PTSD and increased vulnerability to future cognitive impairments. An alternate theory has proposed that cognitive impairment may activate or exacerbate PTSD symptoms that were previously better controlled or less apparent. Floyd, Rice, and Black (2002) suggested that age-related cognitive declines may explain the recurrence of late-life PTSD. Such declines cause an individual to be more prone to intrusive, trauma-related memories, and, coupled with age-related declines in working, episodic, and prospective memory, then raises the level of subjective distress associated with traumatic memories, thus leading to the recurrence of PTSD.

Danckwerts and Leathem (2003) provided a detailed discussion about the limitations of the literature on trauma, PTSD, and cognitive functioning. Much of the current research in this area has been conducted in specific samples (e.g., Caucasian and male veterans), so one needs to be cautious about generalizing to other traumatized populations. Moreover, many of the studies included participants who may meet diagnostic criteria for other disorders in addition to PTSD, which complicates what can be exclusively attributed to PTSD.

It is not yet known what role cognitive impairments may have on the delivery of psychotherapy to older traumatized adults, particularly in CBT interventions, such as PE. Wild and Gur (2008) found that veterans with PTSD, poor verbal memory, and narrative coding impairments were less likely to be responsive to eight sessions of CBT than veterans without PTSD. Those results were maintained even after controlling for intelligence, attention, PTSD severity, depression, time since trauma, and substance abuse.

To date, no scientific literature has indicated that either old age or time since trauma interferes with response to PE (Thorp et al., 2011). It is unclear whether PE will be effective in people with mild, moderate, or severe cognitive impairments. To benefit most from PE, Foa et al. (2007) suggested that a person should have a clear, time-limited memory of a traumatic event. Alternative possibilities for psychosocial intervention in people with moderate to severe cognitive impairment and PTSD are presented elsewhere (Cook, Ruzek & Cassidy, 2003).

DISCUSSION

Although numerous PTSD assessment instruments have fairly good reliability and discriminative validity for use with older combat veterans, little information exists on psychometric properties of those measures in older community-dwelling nonveterans (for a review, see Cook & O'Donnell, 2005). Clearly, more research is needed to determine the reliability and validity of PTSD diagnostic interviews, self-report measures, and screens in the heterogeneous population of older trauma survivors. In addition, psychophysiological and biological assessments may prove a useful and worthy of investigation in this population.

When assessing for traumatic exposure and PTSD in older adults, health care providers need to factor in general considerations. For example, they may consider shame in or fear of reporting traumatic events and associated mental health symptoms, past negative experiences with self-disclosure, inadequate labeling of an event as traumatic or a misunderstanding of terminology, misinterpretation of psychological symptoms as somatic concerns, and aging-related cognitive impairments. Cook and O'Donnell (2005) advised that when assessing older adults for trauma exposure and PTSD, health care providers need to recognize the possibility of multiple lifetime traumas and that symptoms from recent trauma may serve to compound the impact of prior trauma. In addition, PTSD is rarely the sole psychiatric diagnosis, and thus it is imperative to assess for a range of mental health disorders (e.g., depression, substance use disorders).

Providers also must be aware of potential associations between current stressors or developmental milestones and trauma-related symptoms in older trauma survivors. For instance, clinical lore suggests PTSD in older individuals may increase following major life events (e.g., widowhood, retirement, ill health). Another important issue is that initial presentation of PTSD is often less dramatic in older adults, and disclosure of trauma-related symptoms seems to increase after psychoeducation regarding traumatic stress and normalization of related symptoms (Cook & O'Donnell, 2005).

With regard to psychotherapy, although numerous randomized controlled trials have attested to the efficacy of PE, widespread use of exposure therapy for PTSD remains low (Becker et al., 2004; Rosen et al., 2004). Various factors have been hypothesized to account for the lack of exposure use. Client-level variables include complex trauma history or comorbid psychological impairments (e.g., suicidality, self-injurious behaviors); concurrent substance abuse or personality disorders; comorbid psychosocial problems, such as homelessness; declining physical health; inability to disclose trauma history; and treatment noncompliance (Becker et al., 2004; Cook et al., 2005; Litz, Blake, Gerardi, & Keane, 1990). Therapist-level variables, such as inadequate training, low affect tolerance, low levels of confidence in treatment delivery, and previous failure experiences using the treatment can also influence the low use of PE (Litz et al., 1990). Furthermore, therapists may question whether exposing clients to trauma repeatedly, as is required in PE, is revictimizing (Rothbaum & Schwartz, 2002; Zayfert, Becker, & Gillock, 2002) or if treatment needs to be discontinued if the client displays increased anxiety or distress for fear of decompensation (Rothbaum & Schwartz, 2002).

Researchers also have questioned the concern that imaginal exposure may cause symptom exacerbation that leads to premature termination. In a sample of 76 women with chronic PTSD who underwent treatment with PE, only about 10% experienced a temporary PTSD symptom exacerbation, which was unrelated to dropout or outcome (Foa, Zoellner, Feeny, Hembree, & Alvarez-Conrad, 2002). In addition, a review of 25 controlled studies of CBT for PTSD found no difference in dropout rates among exposure and other CBTs, which suggests that PE may not be less tolerable than alternate CBT approaches (Hembree, Foa, et al., 2003).

Numerous modifications can be made to treatment without compromising key elements of the PE protocol. For instance, in the case of a client who is experiencing severe flashbacks or high levels of distress during exposure, the therapist may tell the client to keep his or her eyes open and to switch to the past tense in retelling the trauma narrative; the therapist also may provide grounding comments as the client is retelling the trauma (Hembree, Rauch, & Foa, 2003).

Although client overengagement in therapy may require some modifications, underengagement is generally more common. As the underlying theory of PE posits, PTSD results from excessive cognitive and behavioral avoidance, and underengagement in exposure treatment can be viewed as an avoidant coping strategy to keep from emotionally engaging (Foa & Cahill, 2001). Therapists need to take caution when modifying exposure protocol or integrating elements of various interventions. They may need to make adaptations and can help clients engage safely in exposure therapy. However, some modifications, such as shortening exposure, can actually increase client sensitivity and exacerbate fears (Rothbaum & Schwartz, 2002). Moreover, adding treatment sessions with the intention of preparing clients for PE lengthens the overall program, which may result in increased levels of client dropout.

CONCLUSION

Although PE is highly efficacious, it does not invariably work. Some people do not respond after a full course of PE, and some who complete the therapy experience improvement but remain symptomatic (Foa, 2011). Although exposure therapy is not appropriate for all clients (Foa et al., 2002) and may be particularly difficult to deliver to some populations, preliminary evidence suggests that exposure therapy can be a suitable and effective treatment for cognitively intact older adults with PTSD.

Misguided sympathy on the part of well-intentioned therapists may actually reinforce client avoidance of trauma material and impede emotional processing (Rothbaum & Schwartz, 2002). Although client preference is important in clinical decision-making and likely affects service use and adherence, therapists need to be careful that they do not reinforce clients' maladaptive avoidance. Rarely do clients enter treatment saying, "I want to retell my trauma over and over again," but many do indicate after treatment that such storytelling was a key ingredient in their attainment of symptom reduction (Thorp et al., 2011).

It is possible that empirically minded therapists who may have tried to use PE in their practice without formal training and whose clients may have been reluctant or hesitant, or who experienced symptom exacerbation after their first exposure session, may have led them to abandon or avoid this effective form of treatment. A temporary increase in PTSD symptoms may actually reflect emotional engagement with the traumatic material, which is a positive predictor for successful outcome. Just as safely approaching traumatic memories can build mastery and competence in PTSD clients, so can safely conducting exposure therapy build therapists' confidence and sense of mastery. If therapists are adequately trained, feel competent, and believe in the rationale of exposure, they are likely more apt to effectively deliver PE.

One factor regarding underuse of PE is the relative scarcity of training in its delivery. Over the past several years, the VA has conducted rollouts of two empirically based psychotherapies, PE and cognitive processing therapy, nationally within the VA (Karlin et al., 2010). Those rollouts aimed to ensure permanent capacity to train and supervise mental health practitioners in the delivery of those treatments and to ensure that both become mainstream care in the VA. As part of that dissemination endeavor, a VA intranet website that is accessible only from VA computers (see http://vaww.infoshare.va.gov/sites/PE/default.aspx) assists providers in treatment delivery. The internal VA website offers PE providers a video that can encourage both therapists and clients in the use of this therapeutic form (see http://vaww.infoshare.va.gov/sites/pe/videos/videos.aspx). In addition, the Center for Deployment Psychology offers online and in-person PE training for providers working with veterans and active-duty personnel (see http://deploymentpsych.org/training/online-courses).

Providers outside of the VA health care system interested in PE training can go to http://www.med.upenn.edu/ctsa/workshops_ptsd.html for information on workshops offered by the Center for the Treatment and Study of Anxiety at the University of Pennsylvania. In addition, they may contact Elizabeth Hembree, a codeveloper of PE, for training, supervision, and consultation, by email at hembree@mail.med.upenn.edu or at the Department of Psychiatry, University of Pennsylvania School of Medicine, 3535 Market Street, Suite 600 North, Philadelphia, PA 19104-3309.

REFERENCES

American Psychiatric Association. (2000). *Diagnostic and statistical manual of mental disorders* (4th ed., text rev.). Washington, DC: Author.

American Psychiatric Association. (2013). *Diagnostic and statistical manual of mental disorders* (5th ed.). Arlington, VA: Author.

Asukai, N., Saito, A., Tsuruta, B., Kishimoto, J., & Nishikawa, T. (2010). Efficacy of exposure therapy for Japanese patients with posttraumatic stress disorder due to mixed traumatic events: A randomized controlled study. *Journal of Traumatic Stress, 23,* 744–750. doi:10.1002/jts.20589

Becker, C. B., Zayfert, C., & Anderson, E. (2004). A survey of psychologists' attitudes towards and utilization of exposure therapy for PTSD. *Behaviour Research and Therapy, 42,* 277–292. doi:10.1016/S0005-7967(03)00138-4

Blake, D. D., Weathers, F. W., Nagy, L. M., Kaloupek, D. G., Gusman, F. D., Charney, D. S., & Keane, T. M. (1995). The development of a clinician-administered PTSD scale. *Journal of Traumatic Stress, 8*, 75–90. doi:10.1002/jts.2490080106

Brennan, M., Horowitz, A., & Reinhardt, J. P. (2003). The September 11th attacks and depressive symptomatology among older adults with vision loss in New York City. *Journal of Gerontological Social Work, 40*, 55–71. doi:10.1300/J083v40n04_05

Brown, L. S. (2008). *Cultural competence in trauma theory: Beyond the flashback.* Washington, DC: American Psychological Association. doi:10.1037/11752-000

Cahill, S. P., Rothbaum, B. O., Resick, P. A., & Follette, V. M. (2009). Cognitive–behavioral therapy for adults. In E. B. Foa, T. M. Keane, M. J. Friedman, & J. A. Cohen (Eds.), *Effective treatments for PTSD: Practice guidelines from the International Society for Traumatic Stress Studies* (2nd ed., pp. 139–222). New York, NY: Guilford Press.

Chu, J. P., Huynh, L., & Areán, P. (2012). Cultural adaptation of evidence-based practice utilizing an iterative stakeholder process and theoretical framework: Problem solving therapy for Chinese older adults. *International Journal of Geriatric Psychiatry, 27*, 97–106.

Chung, I. (2003). The impact of the 9/11 attacks on the elderly in NYC Chinatown: Implications for culturally relevant services. *Journal of Gerontological Social Work, 40*, 37–53. doi:10.1300/J083v40n04_04

Coleman, P. G. (1999). Creating a life story. The task of reconciliation. *Gerontologist, 39*, 133–139. doi:10.1093/geront/39.2.133

Cook, J. M., Elhai, J., & Areán, P. A. (2005). Psychometric properties of the PTSD Checklist with older primary care patients. *Journal of Traumatic Stress, 18*, 371–376. doi:10.1002/jts.20038

Cook, J. M., & Elmore, D. L. (2009). Disaster mental health in older adults: Symptoms, policy and planning. In Y. Neria, S. Galea, & F. Norris (Eds.), *Mental health consequences of disasters* (pp. 233–263). New York, NY: Cambridge University Press.

Cook, J. M., & O'Donnell, C. (2005). Assessment and psychological treatment of posttraumatic stress disorder in older adults. *Journal of Geriatric Psychiatry and Neurology, 18*, 61–71. doi:10.1177/0891988705276052

Cook, J. M., Ruzek, J. I., & Cassidy, E. L. (2003). Possible association of posttraumatic stress disorder with cognitive impairment among older adults. *Psychiatric Services, 54*, 1223–1225. doi:10.1176/appi.ps.54.9.1223

Cook, J. M., Schnurr, P. P., & Foa, E. B. (2004). Bridging the gap between posttraumatic stress disorder research and clinical practice: The example of exposure therapy. *Psychotherapy: Theory, Research, Practice, Training, 41*, 374–387. doi:10.1037/0033-3204.41.4.374

Cornelius, T. L., & Kenyon-Jump, R. (2007). Application of cognitive–behavioral treatment for long-standing posttraumatic stress disorder in law enforcement personnel: A case study. *Clinical Case Studies, 6*, 143–160. doi:10.1177/1534650106286544

Danckwerts, A., & Leathem, J. (2003). Questioning the link between PTSD and cognitive dysfunction. *Neuropsychology Review, 13*, 221–235. doi:10.1023/B:NERV.0000009485.76839.b7

Floyd, M., Rice, J., & Black, S. R. (2002). Recurrence of posttraumatic stress disorder in late life: A cognitive aging perspective. *Journal of Clinical Geropsychology, 8*, 303–311. doi:10.1023/A:1019679307628

Foa, E. B. (2011). Prolonged exposure therapy: Past, present and future. *Depression and Anxiety, 28*, 1043–1047. doi:10.1002/da.20907

Foa, E. B., & Cahill, S. P. (2001). Psychological therapies: Emotional processing. In N. J. Smelser & P. B. Baltes (Eds.), *International encyclopedia of the social and behavioral sciences* (pp. 12363–12369). Oxford, England: Elsevier Science.

Foa, E. B., Hembree, E. A., & Rothbaum, B. O. (2007). *Prolonged exposure therapy for PTSD: Emotional processing of traumatic experiences: Therapist guide*. New York, NY: Oxford University Press.

Foa, E. B., Keane, T. M., Friedman, M. J., & Cohen, J. (2009). *Effective treatments for PTSD: Practice guidelines from the International Society for Traumatic Stress Studies* (2nd ed.). New York, NY: Guilford Press.

Foa, E. B., & Kozak, M. J. (1986). Emotional processing of fear: Exposure to corrective information. *Psychological Bulletin, 99*, 20–35. doi:10.1037/0033-2909.99.1.20

Foa, E. B., Zoellner, L. A., Feeny, N. C., Hembree, E. A., & Alvarez-Conrad, J. (2002). Does imaginal exposure exacerbate PTSD symptoms? *Journal of Consulting and Clinical Psychology, 70*, 1022–1028. doi:10.1037/0022-006X.70.4.1022

Friedman, M. J., Resick, P. A., Bryant, R. A., & Brewin, C. R. (2011). Considering PTSD for DSM–5. *Depression and Anxiety, 28*, 750–769. doi:10.1002/da.20767

Gamito, P., Oliveira, J., Rosa, P., Morais, D., Duarte, N., Iliveira, S., & Saraiva, T. (2010). PTSD elderly war veterans: A clinical controlled pilot study. *Cyberpsychology, Behavior, and Social Networking, 13*, 43–48. doi:10.1089/cyber.2009.0237

Golier, J. A., Yehuda, R., Lupien, S. J., Harvey, P. D., Grossman, R., & Elkin, A. (2002). Memory performance in Holocaust survivors with posttraumatic stress disorder. *American Journal of Psychiatry, 159*, 1682–1688. doi:10.1176/appi.ajp.159.10.1682

Hays, P. (2009). Integrating evidence-based practice, cognitive–behavior therapy, and multicultural therapy: Ten steps for culturally competent practice. *Professional Psychology: Research and Practice, 40*, 354–360. doi:10.1037/a0016250

Hembree, E. A., Foa, E. B., Dorfan, N. M., Street, G. P., Kowalski, J., & Tu, X. (2003). Do clients drop out prematurely from exposure therapy for PTSD? *Journal of Traumatic Stress, 16*, 555–562. doi:10.1023/B:JOTS.0000004078.93012.7d

Hembree, E. A., Rauch, S. M., & Foa, E. B. (2003). Beyond the manual: The insider's guide to prolonged exposure therapy for PTSD. *Cognitive and Behavioral Practice, 10*, 22–30. doi:10.1016/S1077-7229(03)80005-6

Himle, J. A., Baser, R. E., Taylor, R. J., Campbell, R. D., & Jackson, J. S. (2009). Anxiety disorders among African Americans, blacks of Caribbean descent, and non-Hispanic whites in the United States. *Journal of Anxiety Disorders, 23*, 578–590. doi:10.1016/j.janxdis.2009.01.002

Hyer, L., Summers, M. N., Boyd, S., Litaker, M., & Boudewyns, P. (1996). Assessment of older combat veterans with the Clinician-Administered PTSD Scale. *Journal of Traumatic Stress, 9*, 587–593. doi:10.1002/jts.2490090314

Hyer, L. A., & Woods, M. G. (1998). Phenomenology and treatment of trauma in later life. In V. M. Follette, J. I. Ruzek, & F. R. Abueg (Eds.), *Cognitive–behavioral therapies for trauma* (pp. 383–414). New York, NY: Guilford Press.

Jaycox, L. H., Foa, E. B., & Morral, A. R. (1998). Influence of emotional engagement and habituation on exposure therapy for PTSD. *Journal of Consulting and Clinical Psychology, 66*, 185–192. doi:10.1037/0022-006X.66.1.185

Karlin, B. E., Ruzek, J. I., Chard, K. M., Monson, C. M., Hembree, E. A., Resick, P. A., & Foa, E. B. (2010). Dissemination of evidence-based psychological treatments for posttraumatic stress disorder in the Veterans Health Administration. *Journal of Traumatic Stress, 23*, 663–673. doi:10.1002/jts.20588

Kruse, A., & Schmitt, E. (1999). Reminiscence of traumatic experiences in (former) Jewish emigrants and extermination camp survivors. In A. Maercker, M. Schützwohl, & Z. Solomon (Eds.), *Post-traumatic stress disorder: A lifespan developmental perspective* (pp. 155–176). Seattle, WA: Hogrefe & Huber.

Lew, L. S. (1991). Elderly Cambodians in Long Beach: Creating cultural access to health care. *Journal of Cross-Cultural Gerontology, 6*, 199–203. doi:10.1007/BF00056757

Litz, B. T., Blake, D. B., Gerardi, R. G., & Keane, T. M. (1990). Decision making guidelines for the use of direct therapeutic exposure in the treatment of post-traumatic stress disorder. *Behavior Therapist, 13*, 91–93.

Mainous, A. G., Smith, D. W., Acierno, R. E., & Geesey, M. E. (2005). Differences in posttraumatic stress disorder symptoms between elderly non-Hispanic whites and African Americans. *Journal of the National Medical Association, 97*, 546–549.

Marsella, A. J., Friedman, M. J., & Spain, E. H. (1992). A selective review of the literature on ethnocultural aspects of PTSD. *PTSD Research Quarterly, 3*, 1–7.

Marshall, R. D., Bryant, R., Amsel, L., Suh, E. J., Cook, J. M., & Neria, Y. (2007). Relative risk perception and September 11th-related PTSD in the context of ongoing threat. *American Psychologist, 62*, 304–316. doi:10.1037/0003-066X.62.4.304

Marshall, R. D., & Suh, E. J. (2003). Contextualizing trauma: Using evidence-based treatments in a multicultural community after September 11th. *Psychiatric Quarterly, 74*, 401–420. doi:10.1023/A:1026043728263

Mays, V. M., Gallardo, M., Shorter-Gooden, K., Robinson-Zanartu, C., Smith, M., McClure, F., . . . Ahhaity, G. (2009). Expanding the circle: Decreasing American Indian mental health disparities through culturally competent teaching about American Indian Mental Health. *American Indian Culture and Research Journal, 33*, 61–83.

Olkin, R. (1999). *What psychotherapists should know about disability*. New York, NY: Guilford Press.

Otto, M. W., Hinton, D., Korbly, N. B., Chea, A., Ba, P., Gershuny, B. S., & Pollack, M. H. (2003). Treatment of pharmacotherapy-refractory posttraumatic stress disorder among Cambodian refugees: A pilot study of combination treatment with cognitive–behavior therapy vs sertraline alone. *Behaviour Research and Therapy, 41*, 1271–1276.

Otto, M. W., & Hinton, D. E. (2006). Modifying exposure-based CBT for Cambodian refugees with posttraumatic stress disorder. *Cognitive and Behavioral Practice, 13*, 261–270. doi:10.1016/j.cbpra.2006.04.007

Paunovic, N., & Ost, L. G. (2001). Cognitive-behavior therapy vs. exposure therapy in the treatment of PTSD in refugees. *Behaviour Research and Therapy, 39*, 1183–1197. doi:10.1016/S0005-7967(00)00093-0

Powers, M. B., Halpern, J. M., Ferenschak, M. P., Gillihan, S. J., & Foa, E. B. (2010). A meta-analytic review of prolonged exposure for posttraumatic stress disorder. *Clinical Psychology Review, 30*, 635–641. doi:10.1016/j.cpr.2010.04.007

Qureshi, S. U., Kimbrell, T., Pyne, J. M., Magruder, K. M., Hudson, T. J., Petersen, N. J., . . . Kunik, M. E. (2010). Greater prevalence and incidence of dementia in older veterans with posttraumatic stress disorder. *Journal of the American Geriatrics Society, 58*, 1627–1633. doi:10.1111/j.1532-5415.2010.02977.x

Renne, J. L., Sanchez, T. W., & Litman, T. (2008). *National study on carless and special needs evacuation planning: A literature review*. New Orleans, LA: University of New Orleans Transportation Center.

Resick, P. A., & Schnicke, M. K. (1993). *Cognitive processing therapy for rape victims: A treatment manual*. Newbury Park, CA: Sage.

Rizvi, S. L., Vogt, D. S., & Resick, P. A. (2009). Cognitive and affective predictors of treatment outcome in cognitive processing therapy and prolonged exposure for posttraumatic stress disorder. *Behaviour Research and Therapy, 47*, 737–743. doi:10.1016/j.brat.2009.06.003

Rosen, C. S., Chow, H. C., Finney, J. F., Greenbaum, M. A., Moos, R. H., Sheikh, J. I., & Yesavage, J. A. (2004). Practice guidelines and VA practice patterns for treating posttraumatic stress disorder. *Journal of Traumatic Stress, 17*, 213–222. doi:10.1023/B:JOTS.0000029264.23878.53

Rothbaum, B. O., & Schwartz, A. C. (2002). Exposure therapy for posttraumatic stress disorder. *American Journal of Psychotherapy, 56*, 59–75.

Russo, S. A., Hersen, M., & Van Hasselt, V. B. (2001). Treatment of reactivated post-traumatic stress disorder: Imaginal exposure in an older adult with multiple traumas. *Behavior Modification, 25*, 94–115. doi:10.1177/0145445501251006

Sachs, G. A., Carter, R., Holtz, L. R., Smith, F., Stump, T. E., Tu, W., & Callahan, C. M. (2011). Cognitive impairment: An independent predictor of excess mortality. *Annals of Internal Medicine, 155,* 300–308. doi:10.7326/0003-4819-155-5-201109060-00007

Schlenger, W. E., Caddell, J. M., Ebert, L., Jordan, B. K., Rourke, K. M., Wilson, D., . . . Kulka, R. A. (2002). Psychological reactions to terrorist attacks: Findings from the national study of Americans' reactions to September 11. *JAMA, 288,* 581–588. doi:10.1001/jama.288.5.581

Strug, D. L., & Mason, S. E. (2007). The impact of September 11th on older Chinese and Hispanic immigrants in New York City. *Journal of Immigrant & Refugee Studies, 5,* 21–44. doi:10.1300/J500v05n02_02

Sutker, P. B., Vasterling, J., Brailey, K., & Allain, A. N. (1995). Memory, attention and executive deficits in POW survivors: Contributing biological and psychological factors. *Neuropsychology, 9,* 118–125. doi:10.1037/0894-4105.9.1.118

Thorp, S. R., Sones, H. M., & Cook, J. M. (2011). Prolonged exposure therapy for older combat veterans in the VA healthcare system. In K. H. Sorocco & S. Lauderdale (Eds.), *Cognitive behavior therapy with older adults: Innovations across care settings* (pp. 421–442). New York, NY: Springer.

Thorp, S. R., Stein, M. B., Jeste, D. V., Patterson, T. L., & Wetherell, J. L. (2012). Prolonged exposure therapy for older veterans with posttraumatic stress disorder: Pilot study. *American Journal of Geriatric Psychiatry, 20,* 276–280. doi:10.1097/JGP.0b013e3182435ee9

Thyer, B. A. (1981). Prolonged in vivo exposure therapy with a 70-year-old woman. *Journal of Behavior Therapy and Experimental Psychiatry, 12,* 69–71. doi:10.1016/0005-7916(81)90032-X

van Zelst, W. H., & Beekman, A. T. F. (2012). Psychometric concerns in the assessment of trauma-related symptoms in older adults. In D. Sloan & J. G. Beck (Eds.), *The handbook of traumatic stress disorders* (pp. 282–301). New York, NY: Oxford University Press. doi:10.1093/oxfordhb/9780195399066.013.0019

Weathers, F. W., Keane, T. M., & Davidson, J. R. T. (2001). Clinician-Administered PTSD scale: A review of the first ten years of research. *Depression and Anxiety, 13,* 132–156. doi:10.1002/da.1029

Weathers, F. W., Litz, B. T., Herman, D. S., Huska, J. A., & Keane, T. M. (1993, October). *The PTSD Checklist (PCL): Reliability, validity and diagnostic utility.* Paper presented at the meeting of the International Society for Traumatic Stress Studies. San Antonio, TX.

Wild, J., & Gur, R. C. (2008). Verbal memory and treatment response in posttraumatic stress disorder. *British Journal of Psychiatry, 193,* 254–255. doi:10.1192/bjp.bp.107.045922

Wolpe, J. (1969). *The practice of behavior therapy.* New York, NY: Pergamon Press.

Yaffe, K., Vittinghoff, E., Lindquist, K., Barnes, D., Covinsky, K. E., Neylan, T., . . . Marmar, C. (2010). Posttraumatic stress disorder and risk of dementia among U.S. veterans. *Archives of General Psychiatry, 67,* 608–613. doi:10.1001/archgenpsychiatry.2010.61

Yoder, M. S., Tuerk, P. W., & Acierno, R. (2010). Prolonged exposure with a World War II veteran: 60 years of guilt and feelings of inadequacy. *Clinical Case Studies, 9,* 457–467.

Zayfert, C., Becker, C. B., & Gillock, K. L. (2002). Managing obstacles to the utilization of exposure therapy with PTSD patients. In L. Vandercreek & T. L. Jackson (Eds.), *Innovations in clinical practice: A source book* (Vol. 20, pp. 201–222). Sarasota, FL: Professional Resource Press.

7

BRIEF ALCOHOL AND DRUG INTERVENTIONS AND MOTIVATIONAL INTERVIEWING FOR OLDER ADULTS

DEREK D. SATRE AND AMY LEIBOWITZ

Alcohol and drug use among older adults is an area of increasing clinical and public health concern. While many adults reduce substance use as they get older, a substantial percentage drink at hazardous levels or use prescription medications or illicit drugs in ways that put them at risk for health problems. As this chapter describes, psychologists have an important opportunity to address this problem through brief interventions and motivational interviewing (MI), which can also be integrated as needed into other mental health services (e.g., treatment of depression) and may serve as an initial step in connecting patients with more extensive alcohol and drug treatment when needed.

This chapter follows the case of "Pablo," an older patient who was referred to a psychologist for evaluation and treatment of depression, poor self-care, and a long history of hazardous drinking. The chapter begins by outlining Pablo's case, along with an introductory description of the brief intervention/MI theoretical approach to addressing problematic alcohol use.

http://dx.doi.org/10.1037/14524-008
Treatment of Late-Life Depression, Anxiety, Trauma, and Substance Abuse, P. A. Areán (Editor)
Copyright © 2015 by the American Psychological Association. All rights reserved.

We also discuss the evidence base for these strategies. A description of how the case was conducted follows next, including discussion of screening, assessment measures, and intervention techniques. The chapter concludes with suggestions for further possible adaptations depending on patient variability in culture, cognitive status, and disability.

INITIAL CASE DESCRIPTION

Pablo is a 68-year-old Mexican American man who retired about a year prior to the time of this referral, after selling the convenience store he owned for many years. Pablo and his wife, Mariana, emigrated from Mexico in their early 20s and had two sons. Mariana died 6 years previously, and Pablo continued to live in the house where he and his wife had raised their family. Their two grown sons lived about an hour's drive away. The older son, Mateo, was married with three young children, and the younger son was single. Pablo's two sisters—and their husbands, children, and grandchildren—also lived in the area.

Pablo was referred to a psychologist by his primary care physician due to concerns about low mood and lack of care for his physical health. Since retiring the year before, Pablo had gained 20 pounds, and his prediabetic condition had progressed to diabetes. He told his doctor that he often let his dog out in the backyard instead of taking her on walks around the neighborhood as he had done previously. He enjoyed occasional visits with his large extended family, but he spent most of his time alone watching television or playing games on the computer.

Pablo had a long history of alcohol use, including what he described as "overdoing it" in adolescence and early adulthood, but he reported cutting back on his drinking after he married. There was also a period, early in his marriage, when Pablo used cocaine regularly. However, he stopped without the aid of any specialized treatment or self-help program when his wife confronted him angrily about his use. During the past few decades, Pablo typically had a beer after work, and sometimes one or two more with dinner. When he was diagnosed with prediabetes a few years ago, he switched to light beer. Since retiring, he started drinking three to four beers most nights, sometimes starting in the afternoon, and sometimes as much as a six-pack. At family gatherings he enjoyed shots of tequila, and he sometimes drank tequila in addition to beer at home by himself. Periodically he has tried to cut back on drinking due to the expense, but over time it creeps back up again.

Pablo also reported to his physician that he suffered from bouts of "low energy" and "feeling down" since the death of his wife 6 years ago. He never spoke with anyone about his sadness and decrease in energy, because he didn't think there was anything unusual about feeling down sometimes and missing his wife. He also felt it was important for him to appear "strong" for his immediate and extended family. He was not aware of anyone in his family ever seeking mental health services. But at the urging of his physician to consider getting help for his low mood and risky drinking, and because of his own worries about his recent diabetes diagnosis, Pablo reluctantly agreed to visit a psychologist.

THEORETICAL BACKGROUND OF MOTIVATIONAL INTERVIEWING

Like many individuals seeking counseling in a mental health setting, Pablo was suffering but had mixed feelings about asking for help and felt unsure about whether it was possible to feel better. He was not sure if anything could help and was uncertain about whether he would be willing or able to make any changes. He was willing to attend therapy because his physician suggested it and because he was worried about the implications of his recent diabetes diagnosis. He admitted to sometimes feeling lonely or sad, but not necessarily "depressed," and did not see a connection between his drinking and his mood and energy level. Pablo's physician may or may not have had time or adequate training to advise Pablo on the impact of alcohol on blood sugar and diabetes. Meanwhile, drinking was one of Pablo's few enjoyable activities, and alcohol was an accompaniment to both relaxation (television and computer games) and family gatherings.

A brief intervention that incorporated MI regarding the risks associated with his current level of alcohol consumption was an appropriate strategy to use with Pablo, and should be considered when therapists are confronted with similar patient circumstances. MI is an ideal approach for engaging individuals who appear unready to make a change or unaware that substance use may be contributing to a variety of problems, including problems with mood, health, and relationships. As designed, MI is a short-term, directive, patient-centered style of counseling that helps clients explore and resolve ambivalence. The therapist actively engages in empathic listening, makes strategic reflective statements that highlight the discrepancy between actual and ideal behavior, and works collaboratively with the client to help increase his or her self-efficacy and intrinsic motivation (Rollnick & Miller, 1995). The therapist's approach involves nonjudgmental guidance and helping the patient increase readiness to change and verbalize intent to change. As further described below, MI is often delivered as part of a brief intervention strategy (typically one to three sessions) and can also be integrated into longer term therapies.

William Miller and Stephen Rollnick (1991) developed MI on the basis of initial work with problem drinkers as part of a general effort to identify "what works" to help enhance behavior change. They linked observations with a number of existing approaches and psychological theories, including Rogers's patient-centered therapy, Bem's self-perception theory, Festinger's theory of cognitive dissonance, and Prochaska and DiClemente's (1992) well-known transtheoretical model of the stages of behavioral change.

Stages of change include *precontemplation*—little or no client awareness of a problem; *contemplation*—a client recognizes a problem and considers whether or not to make a change; *preparation*—a client considers how to change behavior in the near future; *action*—a client actively modifies her or his behavior; and *maintenance*—new patterns of behavior replace old behaviors for an extended period of time.

Acknowledging that change happens in stages, the focus in an MI session is not to "get the client to stop drinking" but to help them move to the next stage of change. Change is usually not a steady, linear process toward improvement; instead, it is typically marked by fluctuating levels of ambivalence, repeated attempts at change, and shifting client goals. MI is a flexible approach that is particularly helpful when working with clients who are in the precontemplation or contemplation phase of change. Miller and Rollnick (1991) further emphasized that (a) ambivalence is normal, (b) change occurs naturally, and (c) the likelihood of change is strongly influenced by relationships—including therapeutic relationships.

The MI model acknowledges that when confronted or coerced, individuals tend to argue, harden their stance, or resist. The more a client articulates a retrenched position (e.g., "alcohol is my only pleasure"), the less likely it is that he or she will change. Most psychologists have encountered the "yes, but . . . " response when a solution or course of action for a client has been suggested too quickly. Clients may spend a great deal of time explaining why the suggested solution won't work or why the problem is not even worth tackling. In contrast to confrontational approaches, which increase resistance, a key goal of MI is to evoke "change talk" from the client. In this approach, the therapist strategically creates a series of opportunities for the *client* to argue for making a change. The theory holds, and evidence supports, that the more individuals verbalize a commitment to change, the more likely they are to actually make that change. MI includes techniques (see the case illustration) that are designed to strengthen or intensify clients' statements of desire, need, ability, and reasons for change—i.e., to strengthen their commitment to change.

At least as important as technique, the overall stance of MI is rooted in Rogerian-style empathy and nonpossessive warmth. MI builds on the idea that the quality of the working alliance between therapist and client is key to therapeutic change, and emphasizes the importance of *accurate empathy*. The therapist facilitates an open exploration of the pros and cons of current substance use, and expresses empathy for the client's dilemma. Accurate empathy enables clients to more fully explore the pros and cons of making a change, which in turn enables a deeper resolution of ambivalence. By evoking and accurately reflecting the client's internal conflict about change versus no-change, and selectively reinforcing change talk, we enable clients to hear themselves in a new light.

A strong evidence base for MI has emerged over the past 20 years. MI has been applied to a range of behavioral health problems (Dunn, Deroo, & Rivara, 2001) and extensively tested for helping individuals decrease or stop alcohol use. It has also been standardized in a number of treatment manuals, is adaptable for use in a variety of healthcare settings (Miller & Rollnick, 2002; Moyers, Martin, Manuel, Hendrickson, & Miller, 2005; Wilk, Jensen, & Havighurst, 1997), and can be delivered in-person and by phone (Cosio et al., 2010; Fleming et al., 2010; Lovejoy et al., 2011). MI has been incorporated into the screening, brief intervention, and referral to treatment (SBIRT) model because it is brief, addresses a range of problem severity, and can enhance patients' motivation to seek substance-use treatment services if needed (Madras et al., 2009).

A small number of studies have examined brief intervention outcomes among older adults, although the content of these interventions was not restricted to MI. In a primary care sample, Fleming (Fleming & Manwell, 1999) compared brief physician advice to reduce drinking to a control group that received a general health booklet. The intervention group had greater reductions in alcohol use. In another primary care study, Blow (Blow & Barry, 2000) found a reduction in consumption and heavy drinking compared with controls. In a controlled trial of 631 adults ages 55 and over recruited in three primary care clinics in Southern California, participants were randomized to receive either a booklet on health behaviors or an intervention condition that included personalized feedback on health behaviors, a drinking diary, and three telephone counseling sessions from a health educator (Moore et al., 2011). At 3 months, fewer intervention group participants reported hazardous drinking. At 12 months, rates of hazardous drinking were not significantly different, although the intervention participants reported fewer drinks in the prior 7 days.

In a study of brief interventions among older adults screened in a range of health and service settings in Florida, prescription medication misuse was the most prevalent substance-use problem, followed by alcohol, over-the-counter medications, and illicit substances (Schonfeld et al., 2010). Depression was prevalent among those with alcohol and prescription medication problems. Those who received a brief intervention had improvement in alcohol and medication misuse, and depression measured at 90-day follow-up interviews compared to baseline (Schonfeld et al., 2010). These studies highlight the efficacy of using brief interventions that incorporate MI techniques.

Brief interventions and MI are especially applicable to older adults because these approaches can be used for patients with a range of alcohol and drug-use patterns. For example, many older adults such as Pablo drink at levels considered risky or problematic, yet may not meet the criteria in the fifth edition of the *Diagnostic and Statistical Manual of Mental Disorders* for a substance use disorder. For example, among adults ages 65 and over who responded to the 2005 National Survey on Drug Use and Health, 13% of men and 8% of women reported at-risk alcohol use (two or more drinks on a usual drinking day within the past 30 days). More than 14% of men and 3% of women in this age group reported binge drinking, defined as five or more drinks, in the past year (Blazer & Wu, 2009). In a large ($N = 5,065$) study of primary care patients ages 60 and over, 15% of men consumed more than 14 drinks per week and 12% of women regularly drank more than seven drinks per week (Adams, Barry, & Fleming, 1996). These prevalence data indicate there are a large number of older adults such as Pablo who could benefit from assistance in cutting back on alcohol consumption.

A number of guidelines have been proposed for screening older adults who may be engaging in risky or hazardous drinking. Screening tools can be used as part of psychologists' initial assessment of older adult clients or in the initial phases of MI to determine whether further exploration of a client's drinking pattern is warranted. Current National Institute on Alcohol Abuse and Alcoholism guidelines recommend that adults over 65 consume no more than three drinks on any one day and no more than seven drinks a week. Based on our case description above, Pablo is clearly drinking more than is recommended.

Older adults such as Pablo are less likely than younger people to seek out formal substance abuse treatment (and such programs may or may not be appropriate for them) but instead come to the attention of health and social service providers (as we see in this case example). For older adults who fall into this category, brief motivational interventions (one to five sessions) focused on health risks and other potential problems associated with drinking may be effective in reducing alcohol consumption (Blow & Barry, 2000). MI can be effective for older adults who engage in hazardous or at-risk drinking (consuming more than is recommended), problem drinking (having adverse consequences), and who may or may not meet diagnostic criteria for a substance use disorder (Blow, 1998). At-risk drinking has also been defined as drinking any alcohol in the presence of certain medical comorbidities, for example, liver disease, pancreatitis, gout, depression, or in combination with medications that could have an adverse interaction (Barnes et al., 2010). For some older individuals with such conditions, any alcohol consumption may be contraindicated.

In thinking about Pablo's circumstances, we can anticipate that he enjoyed drinking, thought of it as a well-deserved reward, a way to dull feelings like loneliness and sadness, and as part of important family celebrations. Most likely he did not know that he was consistently drinking more than is recommended for someone in his age group. He may not have been aware of the potential impact on the future course of his diabetes and his overall health, his mood, and perhaps other problems that he has not discussed yet.

Within the stages of change model, we might think of Pablo as being in the precontemplation stage regarding his understanding of his alcohol use. MI provided a useful framework for exploring with Pablo the pros and cons of his current drinking pattern, in light of his values and goals. The general spirit and specific techniques of MI helped to decrease Pablo's resistance to change and increase his awareness of the role that alcohol played in his life. MI also helped Pablo start to consider whether he would be willing to change his current drinking pattern, and enabled his therapist to provide him with skills and information once he was open to considering these.

CASE ILLUSTRATION

Pablo received four MI sessions with his psychologist in a brief intervention format—one 50-minute in-person session and three 20-minute telephone follow-up sessions. The first session focused on (a) introducing, in a collaborative manner, the idea of discussing Pablo's alcohol use; (b) building rapport using accurate reflections, with particular attention on Pablo's goals and values; (c) briefly engaging Pablo in a discussion about what he liked about drinking, so that he felt understood; (d) evoking negative aspects of drinking (things Pablo was not so happy about, had concerns about, or that moved him away from his goals and values); and (e) summarizing the pros and cons of Pablo's current drinking pattern in a way that highlighted his ambivalence and helped increase his readiness for change. Because Pablo was in a precontemplation stage of change, the emphasis in his initial MI session was on building rapport, encouraging problem recognition, and evoking intrinsic motivation for change.

To orient Pablo to the collaborative nature of the appointment, early in the session the therapist stated, "Your physician mentioned concerns about your health and mood, but I'd like to know what *your* specific concerns are at this time." This type of open-ended question invited him to participate in agenda setting and enabled the therapist to learn more about his values and goals, for example, desire to control his diabetes and perhaps to spend less money on alcohol. It was also important to acknowledge Pablo's ambivalence about therapy and affirm his choice to attend the session, for example, "It can feel uncomfortable to talk with a new person about problems. I appreciate the effort it took for you to come here today." A patient-centered approach to agenda setting enlisted his permission to discuss a topic, such as drinking, that he may or may not have felt was important: "As part of our work together today, in addition to discussing your immediate concerns, I'm going to ask permission to also explore your relationship with alcohol. Would that be OK?"

Miller and Rollnick (2002) identified the basic principles of MI that are key to success with patients such as Pablo: express empathy with the patient's ambivalence around behavior change, develop discrepancy between current behavior patterns and the patient's other goals or values, avoid argumentation, roll with resistance, and support self-efficacy. While some of these, such as "express empathy," may seem like basic counseling skills, it is important to note that with some clients it can be challenging to understand and empathize with their choice to continue drinking (e.g., if the therapist and others believe that drinking is resulting in severe health or psychosocial problems). Other MI principles, such as "rolling with resistance," are departures from earlier styles of confrontation and "breaking through denial." In MI, resistance is seen not as a problematic defense but as a natural reaction to the therapist moving faster than the client (e.g., pushing to the action stage of change when the client is still in contemplation, without taking adequate time for the preparation stage). Signs of resistance (e.g., arguing, ignoring, interrupting) are therefore signals to the therapist to return to an empathic stance, to "come alongside" the client using reflections. When Pablo shared with his therapist in the initial session that he had worked hard since age 16 and had never needed anyone's help, the counselor reflected, "You've always been strong and independent. I would understand if you were hesitant to come here today." Here, the counselor reflected on client strengths and demonstrated acceptance of Pablo's ambivalence right at the outset.

In addition to the overarching principles that characterize MI, Miller and Rollnick (2002) also presented more detailed strategies that help prepare clients for change. These include "opening strategies" that are particularly useful with new clients and those in precontemplation or contemplation stages of change: ask open-ended questions, listen reflectively, summarize, affirm, and evoke self-motivational statements. MI emphasizes open-ended questions ("What do you enjoy about drinking?" and "What are the drawbacks?") and holds that clients should do most of the talking in sessions. MI also acknowledges that too many questions can put clients on the spot, increase defensiveness, and decrease motivation. Careful attention is therefore given to making reflective statements, helping clients to feel understood, and at the same time moving the conversation forward.

As we have already seen, MI includes overarching principles and more specific strategies. A clinician who wishes to become proficient or advanced in MI also learns "microskills" such as specific types of reflections (e.g., amplification) and questions (e.g., looking forward), and a specific MI-consistent style of offering patients information. Although the clinician using MI takes a collaborative stance rather than functioning as an "expert," it is important to provide clients with information that can impact their decision-making. The clinician giving information in an MI-consistent manner asks what the client already knows, reflects that information, and asks permission to share additional information. After sharing a small, critical piece of information, the clinician asks what the client thinks or feels about what was presented. This ask/tell/ask technique respects clients' preexisting knowledge, provides important additional information, and helps clients integrate the new information into their growing understanding.

Pablo mentioned in his initial MI session that he enjoyed drinking and felt it helped him fall asleep at night. However, he also had noticed that lately he had been falling asleep on the sofa more often and was waking up feeling stiff, achy, and unrested. Along with questions, the therapist carefully reflected and summarized Pablo's thoughts, emphasizing the negative aspects of bedtime drinking: "For a while, it seemed like alcohol was helping with sleep, but now your sleep isn't so good. You really want to feel more rested and have more energy." Pablo agreed, and the therapist took this opportunity to offer more information in an MI-consistent manner.

Therapist: What do you know about alcohol and sleep? (ask)

Pablo: Just what I already said—it helps me fall asleep, but sometimes I don't make it to bed.

Therapist: Would it be OK if I shared some information about that? (ask)

Pablo: Sure.

Therapist: Although alcohol can make you sleepy, the quality of that sleep is often poor. This could also increase your risk of injuring yourself in a fall, which is serious as people get older. (tell)

(Pause)

Therapist: What do you make of what I just shared with you?

Pablo: Well, my sleep has been terrible lately. I usually feel pretty steady on my feet, but it's true that when I get up off that sofa in the middle of the night, every muscle in my body aches.

In this case, the therapist offered information that was consistent with Pablo's experience and alerted him to a possible health risk. Pablo responded by considering his experience in a new light, and the therapist guided the conversation toward Pablo's new concerns about pain and injury, and the benefits Pablo has noticed when he drinks less, goes to bed, and gets a good night's sleep.

Miller and Rollnick (2002) stated that change occurs when a person is "ready, willing, and able." MI is a strengths-based approach that enhances not only individuals' motivation to change but also their hope and confidence that they *can* change. For instance, psychologists can support self-efficacy by focusing on previous successes, reframing prior attempts to change, and highlighting skills and strengths that the client already possesses. In Pablo's MI sessions, the therapist continually paid attention to his level of self-efficacy, affirmed his strengths, and noted past successes such as previously quitting cocaine. Past failures to cut back on his drinking were reframed as learning experiences, or practice for future attempts.

It should be noted that although MI is a "structured" brief intervention, it is not scripted, and it requires clinicians to be genuinely empathic and to affirm qualities or skills that they actually see as client strengths. MI is based on the idea that the working relationship between therapist and client is of critical importance, and "faking" empathy or affirmations is unlikely to build a high-quality working relationship. In the case of Pablo, empathy can be developed around the substantial challenges he faces in navigating retirement, adjusting to living alone, the difficulty of giving up an entrenched habit such as daily drinking, or the energy required to increase his activity level when his overall mood is low.

Even when a client feels that a change to their substance-use pattern is important, and that they would be capable of such a change, there may be other priorities in the client's life that get in the way of making an immediate change. This can also be addressed in a motivational interview—usually using a combination of respect for the client's autonomy, and—when appropriate—using MI to highlight the importance of change in a particular area such as substance use.

Brief interventions and MI can benefit from relatively straightforward adaptation for older patients such as Pablo. These include considerations for screening for alcohol use as well as the form and content of the intervention itself (including brief feedback on alcohol use risks as well as MI techniques). As part of the SBIRT public health approach to alcohol screening, it has been recommended that all patients in primary care be screened once per year for hazardous drinking (National Institute on Alcohol Abuse and Alcoholism, 2004). Patients over 65 should be asked whether they had four or more drinks on any one occasion during the prior year (a lower threshold than the five or more drinks used to screen younger adults). This single-item screener has been validated in the general population as a tool for identifying alcohol use disorders. Among slightly longer instruments, the four-item CAGE to screen for lifetime alcohol use disorders (Ewing, 1984) has been validated among older adults. A positive response to one or more CAGE questions should prompt further assessment of a possible current alcohol problem. Comparison of a five-item version of the Alcohol Use Disorders Identification Test (AUDIT; Philpot et al., 2003) versus the full-length version (Babor, Higgins-Biddle, Saunders, & Monteiro, 2001) and the CAGE found that the five-item AUDIT performed as well as the full-length AUDIT and better than the CAGE in identifying alcohol problems among older adults. Thus, the brief AUDIT may be a good choice in health care settings.

For patients with a likely alcohol use problem, the Michigan Alcohol Screening Test—Geriatric Version (MAST–G; Blow et al., 1992) is a screening measure that gives an indication of severity and includes items appropriate to older adults. This scale has 24 items, and five or more positive responses are indicative of an alcohol problem. In developing a brief intervention approach, using these instruments can be helpful in drawing out specific problems that older adults may have encountered from drinking, which may then be incorporated into the therapeutic dialogue.

More broadly, in identifying patients who may benefit from brief interventions, providers working with older patients also should be aware of health issues that could be associated with alcohol or drugs, which should prompt questions regarding possible substance use. These include sleep difficulties, complaints regarding cognitive function, seizures, nutrition issues, liver abnormalities, depression, anxiety, unexplained pain, incontinence, poor hygiene, vision problems, dry mouth, gastrointestinal distress, appetite changes, slurred speech, motor problems, or falls (Blow, 1998). Alcohol or drug use should be considered as a potential contributing factor if any of these problems are present. In our case example, depression is a key presenting issue that alcohol may be contributing to, but there may be additional medical problems linked to alcohol use, such as poor diet and lack of physical activity, that would be worth exploring.

Screening in medical and social service settings is an especially important route for older adults to obtain formal treatment. In our case example, it is very unlikely that Pablo would have sought out treatment to reduce his alcohol problem unless a physician had identified the problem. Targeted screening of older adults in clinical settings where substance abuse prevalence is likely to be high, such as inpatient medical settings, has been the focus of some outreach programs (Satre, Knight, Dickson-Fuhrmann, & Jarvik, 2003). Likewise, the state of Florida's innovative Brief Intervention and Treatment for Elders (BRITE) project (Schonfeld et al., 2010) included screening for alcohol and drug problems in senior centers, clients' homes, and other locations where older adults receive services.

In providing brief interventions and MI to older adults, the medical risks and consequences described here should be conveyed in an empathic, supportive manner that acknowledges the difficulty of cutting back. Some older adults may have greater feelings of guilt or shame regarding drinking or drug use. This sense of shame may be particularly acute among older women drinkers (Wilsnack, Vogeltanz, Diers, & Wilsnack, 1995). Additional cohort effects include greater perceived stigma in seeking out treatment from a mental health professional and reluctance to discuss personal problems with a stranger.

Openly discussing the pros and cons of Pablo's drinking level helped to elicit his own reasons to cut back. After some exploration, it emerged that Pablo's main goals were to have more energy for activities he used to enjoy more—walking his dog, gardening, and spending time with his extended family. Once Pablo became more aware of the negative impact of drinking on his energy level, he became more willing to consider cutting back. Potential courses of action (e.g., self-monitoring with no change, decreasing or moderating his use, a trial period of abstinence) were presented as options, and at each step Pablo chose for himself how to proceed. One follow-up session focused primarily on how to cope with the free-flowing alcohol at family gatherings, and Pablo discovered that as the family elder he was proud to demonstrate to others that he could control his drinking and make healthy choices. Pablo did not find it very difficult to limit himself to one to two drinks per occasion and to decrease his drinking from daily to two to three times per week. However, for clients who are unable to moderate their drinking or who identify abstinence as a goal, the nonconfrontational approach of MI can also facilitate engagement with formal alcohol and drug treatment.

CULTURE, DISABILITY, AND COGNITIVE IMPAIRMENT

By virtue of its client-centered, supportive stance, MI is consistent with culturally competent practice. MI's emphasis on client responsibility and on client–therapist partnership may be more congruent with some cultures than others. MI acknowledges that external circumstances such as social support, financial resources, and access to health care also influence motivation. Fortunately, brief interventions and MI have been just as effective among non-White ethnic groups as among Whites, based on a meta-analysis of MI treatment effects (Hettema, Steele, & Miller, 2005), although such comparisons have not included older adult samples. Similarly, a large multisite study found that brief interventions had comparable efficacy across ethnic groups when examining alcohol and drug use outcomes at 6-month follow-up (Madras et al., 2009). In this study, SBIRT was used in diverse medical settings in six states. Among those individuals reporting baseline illicit drug use, rates of use at 6-month follow-up (measured at four of the six sites) were 68% lower, and heavy drinking was 39% lower. Among those who received brief treatment or were referred to more extensive services, significant improvements were also found in general health and mental health.

Potential differences based on culture include variability regarding the stigma of heavy drinking, extent of family involvement in treatment, or responsibilities to the community. Regardless of ethnic or racial background, it is important to try to understand the client's perspective on alcohol use rather than impose mainstream or dominant-culture values. This, of course, requires knowledge of the influences that promote or sustain substance use among different populations. Motivation-enhancing strategies should be congruent with clients' cultural and social principles, standards, and expectations. For example, older adults often struggle with loss of status and personal identity when they retire (as we see with Pablo), and they may not know how to occupy their leisure time. The impact of this may vary by cultural group. It can be useful to help such retired clients understand their need for new activities and how their use of alcohol may function as a coping mechanism.

There have been few studies examining ethnic differences in older adult drinking patterns and related consequences, which may be relevant in fine-tuning brief intervention approaches. One study comparing African American and White alcohol-dependent men found that African Americans were more likely to have experienced adverse social consequences due to drinking (Gomberg & Nelson, 1995). The authors speculated that once alcohol problems develop, they may become more severe for older minorities due to having fewer financial resources. In addition to cultural and economic factors, ethnic differences in life-course trajectories of alcohol use (Jackson, Williams, & Gomberg, 1998) may be influenced by higher rates of health problems for which drinking is not recommended, such as diabetes, especially among Hispanic and African-American adults (Brancati, Kao, Folsom, Watson, & Szklo, 2000). Thus, providers should be especially alert to the impact of substance problems among older non-White patients and be prepared to integrate health-related information into brief intervention and MI strategies.

Older adults with physical disabilities may require some accommodation in delivering brief interventions and MI. For example, the prevalence of hearing impairment increases with older age (Bovo, Ciorba, & Martini, 2011). Visual impairment also increases with age and has been associated with greater risk for depression (Chou, 2008). In the delivery of brief interventions for alcohol and drug use, psychologists should consider the same type of accommodation for these disabilities that they would use in other forms of psychotherapy, for example, listening assistance devices, or large-print, braille, or audio materials. Content of MI may incorporate the potential for drug and alcohol misuse to exacerbate the impact of a patient's disabilities. For example, patients with mobility problems or visual impairment are at heightened risk of falling, and the therapist can gently introduce this issue into the MI session. For many patients, preventing declines in physical functioning and reducing risk of injury may help motivate them to reduce their alcohol and drug use.

Clinicians also should be aware of possible cognitive impairment among older adults with alcohol and drug problems. There is evidence that cognitive impairment can have a negative impact on alcohol and drug interventions, and it has been associated with lower readiness to change (Blume, Schmaling, & Marlatt, 2005), worse treatment attendance (Copersino et al., 2012), and lower rates of abstinence (Aharonovich, Nunes, & Hasin, 2003). While some cognitive deficits may be transient among older adults and will resolve once substance use stops, others may be long lasting (Draper, Karmel, Gibson, Peut, & Anderson, 2011). If there is any evidence that patients are having difficulty participating in MI treatment sessions due to difficulty in attention, concentration, or memory, conducting a brief cognitive screening is a good idea. One instrument that is sensitive to mild cognitive problems is the Montreal Cognitive Assessment (MoCA; Nasreddine et al., 2005). The MoCA assesses several cognitive domains including attention and concentration, executive function, memory, language, visuoconstructional skills, conceptual thinking, calculations, and orientation. Time to administer the MoCA is about 10 minutes. The total possible score is 30 points, and a score of 26 or above is considered normal. The MoCA instrument, as well as normative data and instructions for use, is available online at http://www.mocatest. org and in most cases can be used free of charge.

If screening suggests cognitive impairment, additional evaluation to diagnose cause and extent of dementia may be warranted. The accurate assessment of the nature and extent of impairment through a neuropsychological evaluation will inform adaptation of the intervention. Strategies for addressing cognitive impairment in adults with more significant alcohol and drug problems include integration of cognitive rehabilitation into detoxification (Goldstein, Haas, Shemansky, Barnett, & Salmon-Cox, 2005) and accommodation based on the extent of impairment. Broadly, to accommodate cognitive changes in some older clients, adaptations may include using a slower tempo of speech, slower pace of therapy, more frequent repetition of material covered to assist in learning, and use of simpler language (Satre, Knight, & David, 2006). These adaptations are relatively simple and apply to other behavioral interventions with older adults as well as to brief interventions and MI. While beyond the scope of this chapter, there are a number of therapeutic strategies to address depression among patients with cognitive impairment that could also be implemented among older adults with co-occurring alcohol and drug use problems, for example, problem-solving therapy or modified cognitive behavioral interventions (Orgeta, Qazi, Spector, & Orrell, 2014; Regan & Varanelli, 2013).

Working collaboratively with family members of older adults with cognitive problems and hazardous drinking should definitely be considered as a way of reducing access to alcohol. Had Pablo shown evidence of cognitive impairment, these types of screening, assessment, and interventions would have been useful.

CONCLUSION

This chapter followed the case of Pablo, a 68-year-old Latino man who reported frequent hazardous drinking, symptoms of depression, and was referred to mental health services from primary care. Other salient aspects of Pablo's situation included his recent retirement and the death of his wife, the new diagnosis of diabetes, and the strong value he placed on strength and independence. A brief intervention incorporated MI approaches and techniques to help him decrease his drinking. Although his medical doctor was primarily concerned with the progression of his diabetes, Pablo became increasingly aware of and motivated by the idea that decreasing his drinking could renew his energy level, increase his ability to engage in enjoyable activities, and even revitalize his position as a role model to his family.

REFERENCES

Adams, W. L., Barry, K. L., & Fleming, M. F. (1996). Screening for problem drinking in older primary care patients. JAMA, 276, 1964–1967. doi:10.1001/jama.1996.03540240042028

Aharonovich, E., Nunes, E., & Hasin, D. (2003). Cognitive impairment, retention and abstinence among cocaine abusers in cognitive-behavioral treatment. Drug and Alcohol Dependence, 71, 207–211. doi:10.1016/S0376-8716(03)00092-9

American Psychiatric Association. (2013). Diagnostic and statistical manual of mental disorders (5th ed.). Arlington, VA: Author.

Babor, T. F., Higgins-Biddle, J. C., Saunders, J. B., & Monteiro, M. G. (2001). AUDIT. The Alcohol Use Disorders Identification Test: Guidelines for use in primary care (2nd ed.). Geneva, Switzerland: World Health Organization, Department of Mental Health and Substance Dependence.

Barnes, A. J., Moore, A. A., Xu, H., Ang, A., Tallen, L., Mirkin, M., & Ettner, S. L. (2010). Prevalence and correlates of at-risk drinking among older adults: The project SHARE study. Journal of General Internal Medicine, 25, 840–846. doi:10.1007/s11606-010-1341-x

Blazer, D. G., & Wu, L. T. (2009). The epidemiology of substance use and disorders among middle aged and elderly community adults: National Survey on

Drug Use and Health. *The American Journal of Geriatric Psychiatry, 17*, 237–245. doi:10.1097/JGP.0b013e318190b8ef

Blow, F. C. (1998). *Substance abuse among older adults. Treatment Improvement Series Protocol (TIP) Series 26*. Rockville, MD: Center for Substance Abuse Treatment, Substance Abuse and Mental Health Services Administration. DHHS Publication No. (SMA) 98–3179.

Blow, F. C., & Barry, K. L. (2000). Older patients with at-risk and problem drinking patterns: New developments in brief interventions. *Journal of Geriatric Psychiatry and Neurology, 13*, 115–123. doi:10.1177/089198870001300304

Blow, F. C., Brower, K. J., Schulenberg, J. E., Demo-Dananberg, L. M., Young, J. P., & Beresford, T. P. (1992). The Michigan Alcoholism Screening Test—Geriatric Version (MAST–G): A new elderly-specific screening instrument. *Alcoholism, Clinical and Experimental Research, 16*, 372.

Blume, A. W., Schmaling, K. B., & Marlatt, G. A. (2005). Memory, executive cognitive function, and readiness to change drinking behavior. *Addictive Behaviors, 30*, 301–314. doi:10.1016/j.addbeh.2004.05.019

Bovo, R., Ciorba, A., & Martini, A. (2011). Environmental and genetic factors in age-related hearing impairment. *Aging Clinical and Experimental Research, 23*, 3–10. doi:10.1007/BF03324947

Brancati, F. L., Kao, W. H., Folsom, A. R., Watson, R. L., & Szklo, M. (2000). Incident Type 2 diabetes mellitus in African American and White adults: The Atherosclerosis Risk in Communities Study. *JAMA, 283*, 2253–2259. doi:10.1001/jama.283.17.2253

Chou, K. L. (2008). Combined effect of vision and hearing impairment on depression in older adults: Evidence from the English Longitudinal Study of Ageing. *Journal of Affective Disorders, 106*, 191–196. doi:10.1016/j.jad.2007.05.028

Copersino, M. L., Schretlen, D. J., Fitzmaurice, G. M., Lukas, S. E., Faberman, J., Sokoloff, J., & Weiss, R. D. (2012). Effects of cognitive impairment on substance abuse treatment attendance: Predictive validation of a brief cognitive screening measure. *The American Journal of Drug and Alcohol Abuse, 38*, 246–250. doi:10.3109/00952990.2012.670866

Cosio, D., Heckman, T. G., Anderson, T., Heckman, B. D., Garske, J., & McCarthy, J. (2010). Telephone-administered motivational interviewing to reduce risky sexual behavior in HIV-infected rural persons: a pilot randomized clinical trial. *Sexually Transmitted Diseases, 37*, 140–146.

Draper, B., Karmel, R., Gibson, D., Peut, A., & Anderson, P. (2011). Alcohol-related cognitive impairment in New South Wales hospital patients aged 50 years and over. *Australian and New Zealand Journal of Psychiatry, 45*, 985–992. doi:10.3109/00048674.2011.610297

Dunn, C., Deroo, L., & Rivara, F. P. (2001). The use of brief interventions adapted from motivational interviewing across behavioral domains: A systematic review. *Addiction, 96*, 1725–1742.

Ewing, J. A. (1984). Detecting alcoholism: The CAGE questionnaire. *JAMA, 252,* 1905–1907. doi:10.1001/jama.1984.03350140051025

Fleming, M., & Manwell, L. B. (1999). Brief intervention in primary care settings. A primary treatment method for at-risk, problem, and dependent drinkers. *Alcohol Research & Health, 23,* 128–137.

Fleming, M. F., Balousek, S. L., Grossberg, P. M., Mundt, M. P., Brown, D., Wiegel, J. R., Zakletskaia, L. I., & Saewyc, E. M. (2010). Brief physician advice for heavy drinking college students: A randomized controlled trial in college health clinics. *Journal of Studies on Alcohol and Drugs, 71,* 23–31.

Goldstein, G., Haas, G. L., Shemansky, W. J., Barnett, B., & Salmon-Cox, S. (2005). Rehabilitation during alcohol detoxication in comorbid neuropsychiatric patients. *Journal of Rehabilitation Research and Development, 42,* 225–234. doi:10.1682/ JRRD.2004.03.0040

Gomberg, E. S., & Nelson, B. W. (1995). Black and white older men: Alcohol use and abuse. In T. P. Beresford & E. S. Gomberg (Eds.), *Alcohol and Aging* (pp. 307–323). New York, NY: Oxford University Press.

Hettema, J., Steele, J., & Miller, W. R. (2005). Motivational interviewing. *Annual Review of Clinical Psychology, 1,* 91–111. doi:10.1146/annurev.clinpsy.1.102803.143833

Jackson, J. S., Williams, D. R., & Gomberg, E. S. L. (1998). Aging and alcohol use among African Americans: A life-course perspective. In E. S. L. Gomberg, A. M. Hegedus, & R. A. Zucker (Eds.), *Alcohol problems and aging* (pp. 63–87). Bethesda, MD: National Institute on Alcohol Abuse and Alcoholism (NIH Publication 98-4163).

Lovejoy, T. I., Heckman, T. G., Suhr, J. A., Anderson, T., Heckman, B. D., & France, C. R. (2011). Telephone-administered motivational interviewing reduces risky sexual behavior in HIV-positive late middle-age and older adults: A pilot randomized controlled trial. *AIDS Behavior, 15,* 1623–1634. doi:10.1007/s10461-011-0016-x

Madras, B. K., Compton, W. M., Avula, D., Stegbauer, T., Stein, J. B., & Clark, H. W. (2009). Screening, brief interventions, referral to treatment (SBIRT) for illicit drug and alcohol use at multiple healthcare sites: Comparison at intake and 6 months later. *Drug and Alcohol Dependence, 99,* 280–295. doi:10.1016/j.drugalcdep.2008.08.003

Miller, W., & Rollnick, S. (1991). *Motivational interviewing: Preparing people to change addictive behavior.* New York, NY: Guilford Press.

Miller, W. R., & Rollnick, S. (2002). *Motivational interviewing: Preparing people for change* (2nd ed.). New York, NY: Guilford Press.

Moore, A. A., Blow, F. C., Hoffing, M., Welgreen, S., Davis, J. W., Lin, J. C., . . . Barry, K. L. (2011). Primary care-based intervention to reduce at-risk drinking in older adults: A randomized controlled trial. *Addiction, 106,* 111–120.

Moyers, T. B., Martin, T., Manuel, J. K., Hendrickson, S. M., & Miller, W. R. (2005). Assessing competence in the use of motivational interviewing. *Journal of Substance Abuse Treatment, 28,* 19–26.

Nasreddine, Z. S., Phillips, N. A., Bedirian, V., Charbonneau, S., Whitehead, V., Collin, I., . . . Chertkow, H. (2005). The Montreal Cognitive Assessment, MoCA: A brief screening tool for mild cognitive impairment. *Journal of the American Geriatrics Society, 53,* 695–699. doi:10.1111/j.1532-5415.2005.53221.x

National Institute on Alcohol Abuse and Alcoholism. (2004). *Helping patients with alcohol problems. A health practitioner's guide.* Retrieved from http://www.csam-asam.org/pdf/misc/PractitionersGuideFINAL.pdf

Orgeta, V., Qazi, A., Spector, A. E., & Orrell, M. (2014). Psychological treatments for depression and anxiety in dementia and mild cognitive impairment. *Cochrane Database of Systematic Reviews, 1,* CD009125.

Philpot, M., Pearson, N., Petratou, V., Dayanandan, R., Silverman, M., & Marshall, J. (2003). Screening for problem drinking in older people referred to a mental health service: A comparison of CAGE and AUDIT. *Aging & Mental Health, 7,* 171–175. doi:10.1080/1360786031000101120

Prochaska, J. O., & DiClemente, C. C. (1992). Stages of change in the modification of problem behaviors. *Progress in Behavior Modification, 28,* 183–218.

Regan, B., & Varanelli, L. (2013). Adjustment, depression, and anxiety in mild cognitive impairment and early dementia: A systematic review of psychological intervention studies. *International Psychogeriatrics, 25,* 1963–1984. doi:10.1017/S104161021300152X

Rollnick, S., & Miller, W. R. (1995). What is motivational interviewing? *Behavioural and Cognitive Psychotherapy, 23,* 325–334. doi:10.1017/S135246580001643X

Satre, D. D., Knight, B. G., & David, S. (2006). Cognitive behavioral interventions with older adults: Integrating clinical and gerontological research. *Professional Psychology: Research and Practice, 37,* 489–498. doi:10.1037/0735-7028.37.5.489

Satre, D. D., Knight, B. G., Dickson-Fuhrmann, E., & Jarvik, L. F. (2003). Predictors of alcohol-treatment seeking in a sample of older veterans in the GET SMART program. *Journal of the American Geriatrics Society, 51,* 380–386. doi:10.1046/j.1532-5415.2003.51112.x

Schonfeld, L., King-Kallimanis, B. L., Duchene, D. M., Etheridge, R. L., Herrera, J. R., Barry, K. L., & Lynn, N. (2010). Screening and brief intervention for substance misuse among older adults: The Florida BRITE project. *American Journal of Public Health, 100,* 108–114. doi:10.2105/AJPH.2008.149534

Wilk, A. I., Jensen, N. M., & Havighurst, T. C. (1997). Meta-analysis of randomized control trials addressing brief interventions in heavy alcohol drinkers. *Journal of General Internal Medicine, 12,* 274–283.

Wilsnack, S. C., Vogeltanz, N. D., Diers, L. E., & Wilsnack, R. W. (1995). Drinking and problem drinking in older women. In T. P. Beresford & E. S. Gomberg (Eds.), *Alcohol and aging* (pp. 263–292). New York, NY: Oxford University.

8

SCREENING, BRIEF INTERVENTION, AND REFERRAL TO TREATMENT (SBIRT) FOR SUBSTANCE ABUSE IN OLDER POPULATIONS

NANCY H. LIU AND JASON M. SATTERFIELD

This chapter describes the screening, brief intervention, and referral to treatment (SBIRT) model for hazardous substance use and substance use disorder (SUD) in older persons. It focuses on strategies to elicit clinically relevant details with important practical steps on how to recognize and prioritize clinical and social sequelae.

Hazardous use (i.e., risky, subsyndromal use) is included in this chapter for conceptual and pragmatic reasons. Conceptually, hazardous use and SUD are understood as a continuum rather than separate diagnostic entities with distinct boundaries (Kendell & Jablensky, 2003). Although not all hazardous users will go on to develop a full-blown SUD, this population is at high risk for a range of medical, psychological, and social injuries. Pragmatically, the hazardous use category comprises the largest population of users seen in primary care and mental health settings (Rigler, 2000). It is imperative to identify these individuals, reduce harm, and prevent progression to a full-blown SUD (Babor et al., 2007).

http://dx.doi.org/10.1037/14524-009
Treatment of Late-Life Depression, Anxiety, Trauma, and Substance Abuse, P. A. Areán (Editor)
Copyright © 2015 by the American Psychological Association. All rights reserved.

We first provide an overview of substance use epidemiology in older populations, including alcohol, illicit drugs, and prescription drug misuse. Second, we present screening and diagnostic considerations, beginning with prescreening questions and continuing to full screening and assessment tools. Last, we highlight special issues for consideration when assessing older adults for SUD and how assessment results shape referral and treatment recommendations.

CLINICAL SCENARIO

Ms. B is a 63-year-old widowed woman with a long history of alcohol misuse and depression. Ms. B was referred by her primary care provider for psychological assessment and possible treatment for alcohol use. Ms. B was hospitalized 2 weeks ago for an upper gastrointestinal (GI) bleed most likely related to alcohol. She followed up at an outpatient primary care clinic after her hospital discharge to monitor the GI bleed and to establish regular medical care. She had no regular primary care provider and had not seen a physician for at least 10 years prior to her hospitalization. This recent hospitalization frightened her enough that she started to think about trying to stop drinking. After leaving the hospital, she abstained from alcohol for 4 days; however, on the fourth day she decided to have one glass of wine with dinner and one glass led to another. Since that time, she is back to drinking on a daily basis, though she has tried to cut down her amount with limited success.

EPIDEMIOLOGY OF SUBSTANCE USE IN OLDER POPULATIONS

Current trends predict that older adults will have greater substance use compared with previous cohorts, and this will be especially true among baby boomers (i.e., persons born between 1946 and 1964; Colliver, Compton, Gfroerer, & Condon, 2006). The prevalence of SUD in the population of those ages 50 years and older is likely to double from 2.8 million in 2002 to 5.7 million in 2020 (Colliver et al., 2006; Han, Gfroerer, Colliver, & Penne, 2009). Although older adults have generally had lower rates of SUD compared with younger adults (Huang et al., 2006; Lin et al., 2011), it is expected that the number of adults ages 50 and older who will need treatment for SUD will increase from 1.7 million in 2000 and 2001 to approximately 4.4 million in 2020 (Gfroerer, Penne, Pemberton, & Folsom, 2003). For use and abuse of illicit drugs, it is expected that treatment needs among persons 50 years and older will increase more than 500% between 1995 and 2020 (Gfroerer

& Epstein, 1999). Especially concerning is the rise in prescription opioid pain relievers across all age groups but especially among older adults (Okie, 2010). In persons ages 65 and over, overdose rates are higher than all other age groups (Dunn et al., 2010).

Alcohol

Among older adults, alcohol is the most abused substance (Gfroerer et al., 2003). Approximately 65% of older adults use alcohol (Blazer & Wu, 2009). In those 50 years or older, 45.1% reported drinking alcohol in the past month (Substance Abuse and Mental Health Services Administration [SAMHSA], 2005). Of these, 12.2% were heavy drinkers and 3.2% were binge drinkers (SAMHSA, 2005). It is estimated that approximately 1% to 3% of adults over 60 in community samples and 10% to 15% of men in medical settings endorse alcohol abuse (Blazer & Wu, 2009). This does not include "at-risk" drinkers who might also benefit from screening and treatment. At-risk drinking was reported in 17% of men and 11% of women ages 50 and over, in 19% of respondents between the ages of 50 and 64 years and 13% of respondents over age 65 (Blazer & Wu, 2009). In those over 50 years, 20% of men and 6% of women reported binge drinking compared with 23% in those between the ages of 50 and 64 and 15% in those older than 65 years.

Demographic patterns among those who abuse alcohol look different among older persons compared with younger persons who abuse alcohol (Atkinson et al., 1990; Schonfeld & Dupree, 1991). Some have estimated that the rate of alcohol abuse among women is about half that of men. Alcohol use tends to be most common among men in the 50-to-64 years age range (Blazer & Wu, 2009).

Older drinkers are usually either new-onset drinkers or lifetime drinkers with accumulated morbidity. Those with new-onset alcohol problems tend to come from higher socioeconomic backgrounds than those who have a younger age of onset. Among these individuals, problematic drinking tends to occur in response to stressors. For example, men who were divorced or separated had a greater likelihood of lifetime alcohol use disorder (Lin et al., 2011). Compared with those with a younger age of onset, there is less family history of alcohol-related problems and fewer psychosocial and legal problems. The frequency and quantity of drinking are less than younger persons who abuse alcohol. Similarly, cognitive problems in those with an older age of onset are less severe and more reversible than those with a younger age of onset (Y. Lee et al., 2010). However, age-associated medical problems not directly related to alcohol abuse, such as hypertension or diabetes mellitus Type 2, may be aggravated by alcohol, and drug-alcohol interactions may pose a more pronounced risk in persons with an older age of onset. Persons with an older age of onset are possibly more compliant with treatment than younger persons who abuse alcohol, and relapse rates do not vary by age of onset.

For lifetime drinkers, the consequences of alcohol use and misuse on older populations can be severe. Given the earlier age of onset, lifetime drinkers are more prone to alcohol-related chronic illnesses (e.g., cirrhosis, pancreatitis, cancers) than those who start drinking in later life (Lin et al., 2011). For these individuals, the consequences of drinking may be greater than for those with a later age of onset, including exacerbation of preexisting medical conditions, cognitive impairment, medication interactions, increased risk of falls, greater social isolation, legal and financial problems, and increased depression and suicide (Satre et al., 2011).

Illicit Drug Use

The baby-boom generation reports higher drug use compared with previous generations (Wu & Blazer, 2011). Drug use is more common among men ages 50 to 64 (Blazer & Wu, 2009). According to the National Survey on Drug Use and Health completed by SAMHSA (2011), of an estimated 4.8 million adults ages 50 and older, approximately 5.2%, reported using an illicit drug in the past year. The most common illicit drug among older adults was marijuana (3.2%), and among those who were over 50 years old, 4% of men and 1.4% of women used marijuana (Blazer & Wu, 2009). Marijuana use is expected to triple between 1999 and 2020 among persons 50 years or older (Colliver et al., 2006). This is also similar to rates in other Western, industrialized nations—in England, lifetime cannabis, amphetamine, cocaine, and LSD use in 50- to 64-year-olds has increased approximately tenfold since 1993 (Fahmy, Hatch, Hotopf, & Stewart, 2012). About 0.8% of older adults reported using another illicit drug, including cocaine (0.6%), heroin (0.1%), hallucinogens (0.1%), and inhalants (0.1%). Among those over 50 years old, 0.73% of men and 0.41% of women used cocaine, and 0.33% met criteria for a drug use disorder (Blazer & Wu, 2009).

Psychoactive Prescription Drugs and Over-the-Counter Medications

Adults ages 65 and older currently consume the most prescription and over-the-counter (OTC) medications compared with other age groups, especially sedatives and opioids (Simoni-Wastila & Yang, 2006; Simoni-Wastila, Zuckerman, Singhal, Briesacher, & Hsu, 2006). Approximately one in four older adults uses medications with abuse potential (Simoni-Wastila & Yang, 2006), and there is a growing rise in their use and abuse. The National

Epidemiologic Survey on Alcohol and Related Conditions defines the non-medical use of prescription drugs as use "without a prescription, in greater amounts, more often, or longer than prescribed, or for a reason other than a doctor said you should use them" (Lin et al., 2011, p. 294). By 2020, the nonmedical use of prescription drugs among adults over 50 years will increase to 2.7 million persons (Simoni-Wastila & Yang, 2006). Lifetime prevalence of nonmedical drug use disorders among persons aged 65 and older is estimated to be 0.6% and past 12-month prevalence was 0.2% (Lin et al., 2011). Among those who are 50 and older, nonmedical use of prescription-type drugs by older adults is 2.3% or 2.1 million users (SAMHSA, 2011). It is estimated that up to 11% of older women misuse prescription medications (Simoni-Wastila & Yang, 2006). Younger age and marital status (i.e., being divorced or separated) were associated with greater odds of lifetime nonmedical use disorder (Lin et al., 2011). Factors associated with this type of abuse include female gender, social isolation, history of SUD or mental health disorder, and medical exposure to prescription drugs with abuse potential (Simoni-Wastila & Yang, 2006). In particular, there is growing use and abuse of prescription opioid pain relievers across all age groups (Okie, 2010), which contributes to the highest mortality for both sexes in people ages 45 to 54 years (Dunn et al., 2010). In people ages 65 and over, overdose rates are higher than younger age groups and similar in men and women (Dunn et al., 2010). Prescription painkillers are the second most prevalent type of abused drug after marijuana (SAMHSA, 2012).

The major classes of prescription drugs with potential for abuse include benzodiazepines, opioids, and stimulants. Benzodiazepines are generally prescribed for anxiety, insomnia, or seizures. Common benzodiazepines include alprazolam (Xanax), chlordiazepoxide, clonazepam (Klonopin), clorazepate, diazepam (Valium), flurazepam, lorazepam (Ativan), oxazepam, and temazepam (Restoril). Even low doses can result in drowsiness, depression, confusion, tremors, and nausea. Long-term effects of the drug include slurred speech, impaired thinking, lack of coordination, confusion, and disorientation. They may cause significant cognitive impairment, which is especially important for older adults. Benzodiazepines are depressants and can slow bodily functions, including breathing and pulse rate. For this reason, it can be extremely dangerous when taken in combination with other depressants, such as alcohol, which could lead to respiratory depression, cardiac arrest, or coma.

Opioids are often prescribed for moderate to severe pain. Acutely, opioids are primarily intended to relieve pain. When chronically administered, however, the intent is to improve social and/or occupational functioning. In general, tolerance to the effects of opioids is common, and chronic pain patients may require complex opioid regimens with escalating doses.

Common Generic Names of Prescription Drugs With Abuse Potential

1. **Benzodiazepines:** alprazolam, chlordiazepoxide, clonazepam, clorazepate, diazepam, flurazepam, lorazepam, oxazepam, temazepam
2. **Opioids:** codeine, dihydrocodeine, fentanyl, hydrocodone, hydromorphone, meperidine, methadone, morphine, oxycodone, oxymorphone, and propoxyphene
3. **Stimulants:** amphetamine, methamphetamine, methylphenidate

Although the majority of patients will not become addicted or misuse opioids, it is important to pay attention to signs of misuse. Overdose can cause respiratory depression and, in some cases, acetaminophen toxicity (e.g., Vicodin, Percocet). Common opioids include codeine, fentanyl, hydrocodone (Vicodin), hydromorphone, methadone, morphine, oxycodone (Oxycontin, Percocet), oxymorphone, and propoxyphene. Intoxication by opioids can include altered mental state, euphoria, sleepiness, and poor attention, alternating with withdrawal symptoms, including nausea, muscle/joint pain, diaphoresis, tremor, anxiety, restless, cravings, and poor attention. Opioids can also interact with alcohol, benzodiazepines, and antihistamines. Signs of dangerous combinations may include trouble breathing, weakness, confusion, and anxiety or severe drowsiness and dizziness.

Prescription stimulants are typically used for attention problems or general alertness. Common drugs include amphetamines, methylphenidate (Ritalin), and methamphetamine. Possible misuse may include use for weight management or recreational use. Side effects may include sweating, nervousness, insomnia, frequent urination, and increased risk for cardiovascular problems, such as heart attack and stroke. For a summary of prescription drugs with abuse potential, see Exhibit 8.1.

Tobacco

Nicotine dependence is an SUD resulting from chronic tobacco use. Smoking is responsible for more medical morbidity and mortality than all other SUDs combined. Tobacco use often co-occurs with alcohol and/or drug use, and smoking prevalence rates are higher in patients with mental illness. Older adults may have started smoking long before current public health efforts to educate the public and may—erroneously—feel less motivated to quit since "the damage is already done." Nicotine dependence should be screened, assessed, and treated as any other addiction and need not be "tolerated" while a patient works on other comorbid problems. Several high-quality tobacco cessation resources are readily available (Fiore et al., 2008).

SPECIAL CONSIDERATIONS FOR SUBSTANCE ABUSE AMONG OLDER POPULATIONS

The physical, psychological, and social vulnerabilities of older persons contribute to the unique challenges of assessing substance use in this population. Tolerance is affected by the aging process. Patients may experience increased sensitivity to substances, which may cause problems even with low intake (e.g., higher blood alcohol levels than younger persons who consume the same amount of alcohol; SAMHSA, 1998). They often have chronic medical conditions that amplify the consequences of use. For example, gastrointestinal disease and bleeding are common reasons for emergency department visits by older adults with alcohol problems (Adams, Magruder-Habib, Trued, & Broome, 1992). Medications used to treat chronic conditions (or medications in general) can interact with substances, like alcohol or illicit drugs, altering efficacy or causing physical harm (e.g., Pringle, Ahem, Heller, Gold, & Brown, 2005). For example, combining alcohol and sedatives can depress respiration and result in death. Alcohol and drug clearance slow with age, which can increase intoxication and likelihood of overdose and medical complications (Moos, Brennan, Schutte, & Moos, 2004; Vestal et al., 1977). Psychologists should consult electronic health records and directly communicate with primary care providers for a thorough medical and medication history. It is necessary to educate patients about the risks of drug interactions and monitoring for proper dosage and scheduling intervals. Long-term drinkers and/or drug users in particular may need to learn about these physical changes and lower limits of safe use.

Hazardous use and SUD are often complicated by co-occurrence with psychological problems, such as major depression (Davis, Uezato, Newell, & Frazier, 2008). This combination of substances and mental health problems presents a high risk factor for suicide in Europe and North America (World Health Organization Suicide Prevention [SUPRE], 2012). Older adults constitute the demographic group with the highest suicide rates for most countries in the world (WHO, 2012). Substances can be both causes and effects of mental health problems (Cook, Winokur, Garvey, & Beach, 1991; Saunders, et al., 1991).

Social factors also affect use in this population. Poverty rates are higher for older people than the population as a whole (Organization for Economic Cooperation and Development, 2011). Income maintenance and finances may be stressful. Ageism (i.e., feeling less valued and invisible to society) can cause "minority" stress. Bereavement, especially loss of friends or a significant other, is common and may contribute to depression and isolation. Distance from younger family members and friends may exacerbate these feelings.

Finally, older persons tend to be reluctant to seek treatment and may hold negative beliefs about treatment and mental health providers. Stigma can prevent older persons from seeking treatment and once in treatment, underreporting can result from shame, mistrust, or social desirability. Older adults prefer to seek help from primary care clinics rather than mental health specialty clinics and consultation with medical providers may lessen the stigma associated with seeking mental health treatment.

Management of Substance Use

Given the concern regarding the prevalence of substance use in older persons, two leading models offer suggestions on how substance use should be managed within a medical setting—the classic 5As model that first originated with smoking, and a newer SBIRT model that refers to the steps of Screening, Brief Intervention, and Referral to Treatment. Although designed for traditional medical settings, these models provide useful information for the assessment and management of SUD, especially when a mental health professional might play an important role.

The U.S. Preventive Services Task Force (USPSTF; 2012) described the 5As behavioral framework for use as an alcohol screening tool: (1) Assess alcohol consumption with a brief screening tool followed by clinical assessment as needed (particularly physical health consequences and comorbid mental health problems, if any); (2) advise patients to reduce alcohol consumption to moderate levels; (3) agree on individual goals for reducing alcohol use or abstinence (if indicated); (4) assist patients with acquiring the motivation, self-help skills, or support needed for behavior change; and (5) arrange for follow-up support and repeated counseling, including referring dependent drinkers for specialty treatment. Common successful interventions include motivational interviewing (see Chapter 7, this volume). Additional screening tools, updates, and copies of screening tools are available at the National Institute on Alcohol Abuse and Alcoholism (NIAAA) website: http://www. niaaa.nih.gov/.

Screening, Brief Intervention, Referral, and Treatment: Theoretical Background and Application to Aging

SBIRT (Schonfeld et al., 2010) is a comprehensive, integrated, public health approach to the delivery of early intervention and treatment services for persons with SUD, as well as those who are at risk of developing these disorders. Primary care centers, hospital emergency departments, trauma centers, and other community health settings provide opportunities for early intervention with at-risk substance users before more severe consequences occur. Screening quickly assesses the severity of substance use and identifies the appropriate level of treatment. SBIRT is an evidence-based intervention strategy developed and tested in emergency and internal medicine departments (Babor, et al., 2007) that is applicable to a wide range of health settings. In a multisite study in which over 450,000 patients were screened, those who received a brief intervention had significant declines in heavy alcohol use (38.6% decrease) and illicit drug use (67.7% decrease) at 6-month follow-up, and those who received specialty care reported significant improvements in general health, mental health, employment, housing status, and criminal behavior (Madras et al., 2009). A recent meta-analysis of randomized controlled trials and cost-effectiveness studies showed that SBIRT is one of the top five highest impact preventive interventions, on par with screening for hypertension or influenza vaccinations (Maciosek et al., 2006; Solberg, Maciosek, & Edwards, 2008).

SBIRT can be very brief (e.g., 5–10 minutes in emergency department settings) and may use a variety of motivational interviewing skills to facilitate reliable assessments, brief interventions to reduce use or harm, and referrals to specialty care if needed. Mental health providers may enter into the SBIRT process in a number of important ways. First, integrated behavioral health providers may do the initial screening and in-house brief interventions or provide structured brief treatment. Even if the services are not directly provided by the mental health professional, he or she may serve in an important consultative role to the primary care provider and clinic staff. Mental health providers may also be on the "receiving end" of the "RT" aspect of SBIRT by providing specialty care for SUD and potentially collaborating with the referring providers to best coordinate care. Last, mental health providers are well positioned to perform in-depth assessments, make specialty care referral recommendations, and prepare the patient to accept a referral. We describe the process of screening and assessment for each substance of abuse and then return to the opening clinical case.

Prescreening and Screening

Hazardous use and SUD use often go undetected or underreported in older adults. Providers may confuse signs of SUD with age-related changes, such as cognitive decline, psychomotor retardation, depression, weight loss, or GI conditions. Misperceptions about the low prevalence of SUD among older adults may also lead clinicians to dismiss the possibility of SUD. Patients may experience shame and guilt and seek to conceal substance abuse problems, or providers may be reluctant to ask.

However, the benefits of early and accurate identification of hazardous use and SUD clearly outweigh the risks. Evidence-based models reveal significant success and can prevent further complications from use. Also, older adults typically display high SUD treatment attendance, compliance, and response, which highlight the value of early identification and connection with treatment (Lemke, & Moos, 2003; Oslin, Pettinati, & Volpicelli, 2002).

Prescreening and screening are the first steps in determining current substance use and associated risks. *Prescreening* consists of highly sensitive questions that are often asked by medical providers. *Screening* is a brief process that identifies individuals who have or are at high risk for an SUD. Screening prioritizes domains that require further assessment and is an essential component of a comprehensive and thorough evidence-based assessment. The USPSTF (2012) recommends universal, annual alcohol screening in primary care. Unfortunately, patients are often not screened or those identified as at-risk are not followed up with appropriately (Friedmann, McCullough, Chin, & Saitz, 2000). Although there are no current USPSTF recommendations for universal illicit drug use screening, we recommend that all therapy patients be screened for SUD even if they were not specifically referred for that reason.

A universal prescreening instrument is often used to identify patients who potentially fall into one of the problematic categories. Prescreening questions are highly sensitive and should only be used to selectively identify those patients who require further screening. Although prescreening is usually done before the patient is referred to a mental health provider for further assessment, these prescreening questions are included below in the relevant substance-related section. Prescreenings often dictate which patients receive a full screening instrument.

Screening is distinct from diagnosis because its goal is to identify individuals who have a high probability of having or developing the disorder and/ or associated complications. Positive scores on full screeners indicate the need for a thorough clinical assessment. The following provides a brief overview of prescreening questions, evidence-based screening tools, and recommended assessment content for alcohol, illicit drugs, and prescription drug abuse.

Alcohol Screening Tools

Primary care clinics most commonly use the NIAAA single question prescreener that asks about binge drinking, "How many times in the past year have you drank five (men) or four (women) drinks or more in one day?" Any answer greater than zero (for a patient of any age) indicates that this patient is potentially at risk and should be given a full screener. Primary care clinics may follow-up with basic frequency and quantity questions: "On average, how many days per week do you drink? On those days, how many drinks do you typically have?" Moderate drinking is defined as no more than 14 drinks/week (or two per day on average) for men and seven drinks/week (or one per day on average) for women. Drinking above these moderate limits places the patient at risk and indicates the need for a full screen and possible intervention. It is important to note that the definitions of moderate drinking and binge drinking change at age 65. For older adults (ages 65 and over), moderate drinking is redefined as one standard drink or less per day (seven per week) for men and one drink or less per day (seven per week) for women (USPSTF, 2012). Binge drinking is defined as four or more drinks in one day for both men and women 65 and older.

Although mental health providers (and third-party payers) often think in terms of diagnostic entities such as alcohol abuse or alcohol dependence, it is critical to recognize and appreciate the larger category of risky or hazardous drinking often detected by sensitive prescreening. Hazardous use is characterized by physical, social, or psychological harm from alcohol use without meeting criteria for abuse or dependence (USPSTF, 2012).

Most patients referred to a mental health provider will have already scored positive on a substance use prescreen. Full screening tools can gather additional information helpful in further classifying use patterns and risk. These tools may also be used for repeated measures to assess disease progression over time or the effectiveness of treatment interventions. We briefly describe several commonly used alcohol screeners below.

- Alcohol Use Disorders Identification Test (AUDIT; Babor, Biddle-Higgins, Saunders, & Monteiro, 2001; Saunders, Aasland, Babor, de la Fuente, & Grant, 1993): This instrument consists of 10 brief questions scored on a 0-to-4 rating scale where scores lower than 8 indicate a strong likelihood of hazardous alcohol consumption and scores greater than 16 are a strong indicator for alcohol abuse or dependence and should trigger a full assessment with possible referral to treatment. This test is one of the most studied screening tools for detecting alcohol problems in primary care and is sometimes used in a three-item prescreen version called the AUDIT–C. The 10-item AUDIT has demonstrated sensitivity for detecting harmful alcohol use and abuse or dependence. Research is underway to use the AUDIT in a web-based format (Kypri, Langley, Saunders, Cashell-Smith, & Herbison, 2008).
- Alcohol, Smoking, and Substance Involvement Screening Test (ASSIST; World Health Organization ASSIST Working Group, 2002). This is a lengthier and more comprehensive assessment that was developed by an international group of substance abuse researchers to detect and manage all substance

use and related problems in primary and general medical care settings. Although its length precludes use in primary care settings, it could prove useful in longer, more in-depth mental health visits. The ASSIST is available in English and 10 other languages. A copy of the assessment is available at http://www. who.int/substance_abuse/activities/assist_v3_english.pdf

- CAGE: Cut down, Annoyed, Guilty, Eye opener (Ewing, 1984). CAGE consists of just four questions in yes/no format. If a patient has two or more yes answers, this indicates a possibly significant alcohol problem. This traditional assessment is still commonly taught in medical schools and remains popular in primary care settings despite somewhat mediocre psychometrics and limited utility in measuring severity or treatment progress (Ewing, 1984). CAGE is sometimes used as a prescreening tool that is then followed up with by the AUDIT or ASSIST.

Illicit Drugs

As with alcohol, medical clinics often use a single item drug-screening question: "How many times in the past year have you used an illegal drug or used a prescription medication for nonmedical reasons?" This question has demonstrated high sensitivity but limited specificity (Smith, Schmidt, Allensworth-Davies, & Saitz, 2010). Although this single-item screener is widely used, there is limited evidence of its appropriateness for older adults. Alternatively, the Two-Item Conjoint Screen (TICS; Brown et al., 2001) targets both alcohol and drug use. The two questions are: "In the last year, have you ever drunk or used drugs more than you meant to?" and "Have you felt you wanted or needed to cut down on your drinking or drug use in the last year?" At least one positive response detected current SUD with nearly 80% sensitivity and specificity. There is some evidence that the TICS demonstrates adequate psychometric properties among a variety of patients presenting at an urban primary care centers, including older adults (J. D. Lee, Delbanco, Wu, & Gourevitch, 2011).

The original Drug Abuse Screening Test (DAST; Skinner, 1982) is a 28-item yes/no format measure that uses self-report of consequences or problems related to drug use that are combined to obtain a total score ranging from 0 to 28. This score represents a quantitative estimate of problems associated with drug use and demonstrates good concurrent and discriminant validity, as well as good reliability and internal consistency (Gavin, Ross, & Skinner, 1989; Yudko, Lozhikina, & Fouts, 2007). A cutoff score of 6 indicates drug misuse with adequate sensitivity and specificity (Yudko et al., 2007). It should be noted that shorter versions of 20 (DAST–20) and 10 items (DAST–10) have been developed and validated showing nearly equivalent test characteristics as the longer version (Yudko et al., 2007). The cutoff score for the DAST–10 is typically 3. Since the patient must repeat all of the questions for each drug being used, it is particularly helpful to use shorter versions when polysubstance use is suspected.

Prescription Drugs and Over-the-Counter Medications

Recent clinical guidelines recommend that treating chronic pain with opioids should include monitoring with urine drug testing, frequent prescriber visits, pill counts, and use of state prescription drug monitoring program data (Liebschutz & Alford, 2011). For this reason, communication and consultation with physicians may provide the most accurate information regarding the harm or misuse of these drugs. In general, psychologists should remember that good pain management should lead to some decrease in perceived pain combined with a corresponding increase in an ability to function (Passik & Kirsch, 2008). Typically, the prescreen used for illicit drugs includes the prescreen for prescription drug abuse: "How many times in the past year have you used an illegal drug or used a prescription medication for nonmedical reasons?" If necessary, "nonmedical reasons" can be clarified as using prescription medications "because of the way they made you feel" or "in a way other than as prescribed by your doctor." Technically, this includes the use of another person's medication even if the use is later deemed medically appropriate.

There are a limited number of screening measures for prescription drug abuse or OTC medication misuse. A useful clinical pearl when looking for a potential prescription drug abuse problem is the 4 Cs: (1) loss of control, (2) compulsive use, (3) continued use despite harm, and (4) craving. The following are several commonly used prescription drugs and OTC medications screeners.

- Potential Aberrant Drug-Related Behavior and Assessment (Fleming, Davis, & Passik, 2008; Passik & Kirsh, 2004). This measure identifies four behaviors—over-sedating oneself, feeling intoxicated, getting early refills, increasing dosage on own—that predict patients at greatest risk for a current SUD. Patients who report four or more aberrant drug behaviors are associated with a current SUD and illicit drug use, whereas those with up to three aberrant behaviors have very low probability of a current SUD.
- Screener and Opioid Assessment for Patients with Pain—Revised (SOAPP–R; Butler, Budman, Fernandez, & Jamison, 2004; Butler, Fernandez, Benoit, Budman, & Jamison, 2008).

This 14-item measure identifies chronic pain patients who may be at risk for problems with long-term opioid medication use. Studies show internal reliability and predictive validity with other measures. Items include questions about stress management, medication behaviors, and past drug problems. A copy is available at http://www.painedu.org/soap.asp.

- Current Opioid Misuse Measure (COMM; Chou et al., 2009). This is a 40-item self-report assessment of past-month aberrant medication-related behaviors, defined as those that are concerning for addiction or taking medication other than how it is prescribed. It focuses on actual medication use over the past month rather than risk potential for abuse. Using a score of greater than or equal to 13, this measure demonstrates adequate sensitivity and specificity for an actual *DSM–IV–TR* prescription drug use disorder (Meltzer et al., 2011). It is available at http://www.painedu.org/soapp.asp.

Prescreening and Screening for Ms. B

Ms. B arrived at her appointment with her therapist, who reviewed the prescreening done in the primary care clinic and conducted a full screen using the AUDIT. In response to the NIAAA single-question prescreener about binge drinking ("How many times in the past year have you drank four drinks or more in one day?"), Ms. B reported that she drank four drinks per day nearly every day. When asked, "How many times in the past year have you used an illegal drug or used a prescription medication for nonmedical reasons," Ms. B admitted to smoking marijuana as a young adult but denied any drug use in the past year. The therapist administered the AUDIT to assess the severity of her drinking. Ms. B scored 18, with frequent binges and blackouts. Her score of 18 placed her in the severe or "probably dependent" category. The therapist continued with a full assessment.

CLINICAL ASSESSMENT

After relevant screenings have been completed, indicated individuals should receive an in-depth clinical assessment. Whereas screening is the process of evaluating whether there is a substance problem, assessment is the process of defining the nature of the problem, determining a diagnosis, and developing specific treatment recommendations for addressing the substance problem. There are three main goals of assessment: (1) determine whether the individual meets criteria for a diagnosis;

(2) understand the details regarding the frequency, intensity, duration and functional impact of use, and important behavioral and psychosocial contextual factors that affect use; and (3) use gathered clinical assessment information for the selection of appropriate treatment interventions to address the identified problems. Specific techniques and algorithms for brief interventions, referrals, and treatment are provided in subsequent chapters.

DSM–5 Criteria for Substance Use Disorder

The first goal of a clinical assessment is to establish whether the patient meets criteria for a diagnosis, noting that the absence of a diagnosis does not preclude a referral to treatment. If the patient does not meet criteria for an SUD, it is still necessary to conduct an assessment of subthreshold or hazardous use. Those endorsing potentially harmful use and more developed SUD problems should be periodically reassessed to determine if DSM criteria have been met. Most of the assessment questions are similar across substances and fall into the broad categories of diagnosis in accordance with the fifth edition of the *Diagnostic and Statistical Manual of Mental Disorders* (*DSM–5*; American Psychiatric Association, 2013). In contrast to *DSM–IV–TR* (American Psychiatric Association [APA], 1994), *DSM–5* includes a reorganization of abuse and dependence into one disorder of graded clinical severity where two criteria are required to make a diagnosis (American Psychiatric Association, 2013). In *DSM–5*, craving has become a new criterion and the legal problems criterion has been removed. The sections that follow describe the major assessment domains mental health professionals should consider; Exhibit 8.2 summarizes those plus additional domains to explore, depending on the screening results.

EXHIBIT 8.2
Major Assessment Domains for Substance Abuse Disorder

Current Use
1. Frequency/quantity
2. Duration/pattern of use
3. Route of administration
4. Readiness to change
5. Triggers, obstacles/facilitators

Historical Factors
1. Past quit attempts
2. Past treatment
3. Past medical history
4. Family history of SUD

Contextual Factors
1. Current medical problems
2. Comorbid mental health conditions
3. Socioeconomic status
4. Social supports
5. Living situation
6. Resources

Note. SUD = substance use disorder.

Functional Impairment

All SUD diagnoses require the presence of social and/or occupational functional impairment. In the absence of a diagnosis, a thorough understanding of functional impairment is also necessary to understand the problems associated with use, including hazardous use. Functional impairment can be assessed by examining activities of daily living (ADLs), instrumental activities of daily living (IADLs), and advanced activities of daily living (AADLs). Basic ADLs include bathing, dressing, going to the toilet, continence and feeding, and other behaviors that a person cannot avoid in a day's routine. Questions might include "Are you able to dress and undress without help?" These queries might be further broken down into key steps. With dressing, for example, questions might focus on the ability to deal with buttons, zippers, or similar fastener without external help. IADLs are activities that require more cognitive abilities and include shopping, using transportation or driving, being responsible for taking medications, cooking, doing housework, doing laundry, and managing finances. AADLs include the ability to engage in hobbies, socialize, volunteer or work, or do other patient-specific recreational activities. Detection of problems depends on baseline activity levels and older adults in general may be engaged in fewer activities than younger persons, making detection of problems difficult. Many older adults may be retired from their primary employment, for example, and in these instances, occupational impairment should be broadened to include volunteer work, hobbies, or having trouble with ADLs as a consequence of substance use.

Functional impairments can be assessed with the Kohlman Evaluation of Living Skills (KELS; Kohlman-Thomson, 1992), Katz Index of Independence in Activities of Daily Living (Katz ADL; Katz, Ford, Moskowitz, Jackson, & Jaffe, 1963), Independent Living Scales (ILS; Loeb, 1996), or asking specific questions regarding ADLs. Social impairments may be captured within AADLs but signs of impairment might also include frequent conflict with family or friends (often around substance use), loss or dissolution of relationships, emotional distance from adult children, not being allowed to be with grandchildren when unsupervised, and social or sexual problems.

By definition, appropriate prescription and OTC drug use should result in functional improvement whereas misuse should cause functional impairment. Assessment should compare the intended goal of the medication with its actual impact on functioning as defined in concrete, behavioral terms (e.g., ability to shower, go grocery shopping). For example, pain medications should sufficiently lower pain to allow the patient to reengage with typical daily activities without causing excessive drowsiness, memory impairment, or detachment from family and friends (e.g., pain medications should allow an individual to return to work and not need to call in sick).

Assessing Medical Comorbidities

With ongoing changes to the health care system, it is increasingly important for psychologists to closely collaborate with primary medical providers and to become more integrated within interdisciplinary health-care teams. Especially with SUD, there are significant comorbidities, drug interactions, urinary toxicology and other laboratory results, and additional health information that should be considered when assessing and treating a patient. Considering the various health concerns of older populations, psychologists should obtain a release of medical information to facilitate communication between mental health and primary care providers. Assessments in this category begin with the medical record and should continue with discussions including both the primary care provider and the patient. Baseline medical comorbidities and their current level of severity should be documented so future changes can be more easily noted.

Since patients typically see their mental health provider more often than their primary care provider, mental health practitioners are ideally situated to note and report ongoing changes in health status. For example, patients with alcohol use disorders may report exacerbations with dyspepsia, insomnia, peptic ulcer disease, pancreatitis, esophageal varices, or vasculitis—all important information for a primary care provider to know. Similarly, mental health providers may be the first to learn about alcohol-related falls, accidents, blackouts, or other indicators of possible medical or neurologic harm.

Psychosocial/Behavioral Assessment of Substance Use

It is important to assess the specific patterns and social contexts associated with substance use. Assessment should focus on the type of substance, duration of use, frequency of use, and route of administration. Questions might include open-ended questions regarding use, such as "How often do you drink?" Another useful technique is to start with the question "When was the last time you drank?" and subsequent questions can be an entryway to more information about how the most recent use compares with typical use. Although much of this information may have been captured in the prescreen or screening process, additional information on readiness to change, triggers, facilitators, inhibitors, supports, and resources can prove helpful when planning and delivering treatment. Sample questions might include "What was helpful for you the last time you were able to cut down on your use?" and "Can you think of anything that might make cutting down more difficult?" Important historical factors include past quit attempts, details of past SUD treatment, family history of SUD, past medical conditions related to substance use, and current comorbid medical or psychiatric problems. Social contextual factors include current socioeconomic status, living situation, social supports, and substance use patterns of important individuals in the patient's social network. We will illustrate how this works by revisiting our clinical illustration.

Other Sources of Assessment Information

In addition to the more traditional intake interview, several other resources provide useful information for psychologists working with an older patient with hazardous use or an SUD.

- *Collateral contacts.* For patients living in assisted-living facilities, with family or with cognitive impairments, collateral information regarding substance use and functional impairment can provide useful additional information that may not be provided directly from the patient. Of course, patients must give their consent if confidential health information is to be shared. Moreover, developing a sense of a patient's social network and quality of social supports may provide important insights into their substance use behavior and possible supports for treatment.
- *Urinalysis/urine toxicology.* In addition to self-report behavioral information, point-of-service or laboratory urine tests might serve as an important part of screening, especially when questions remain about actual use of the substances in question. A point-of-care test (POCT) is a drug or validity test conducted at the collection site to obtain an initial or screening result on whether a specimen contains a drug or drug metabolite or is not a valid specimen. It is also called onsite, point-of-service, or point-of-collection test (SAMHSA, 2011). Screening POCT devices are available for urine and oral fluids (saliva). A POCT is a screening test, and a confirmatory drug test is usually more technically complex. According to the SAMHSA treatment improvement protocol (Blow, 1998), the practitioner can decide whether to request a confirmatory test:

    When a patient's screening test (either a POCT or laboratory test) yields unexpected results (positive when in SUD or negative if in pain management treatment) the practitioner decides whether to request a confirmatory test. In addition, a confirmatory test may not be needed; patients may admit to drug use or not taking scheduled medications when told of the drug test results, negating the necessity of a confirmatory test. However, if the patient disputes the unexpected findings, a confirmatory test should be done.

POCTs are well-established, rapid, inexpensive, and simple for drug detection (Watson et al., 2006). Most laboratories use established cutoffs. A urinalysis or urine toxicology screen can be useful for identifying use of certain substances or determining whether prescription medications are being used as prescribed. In fact, for patients on chronic opioids, it is considered a standard of care to order periodic urine drug screens. These screens ensure that opioids are being taken but also test for concurrent use of illicit drugs. Psychologists working in primary care settings might consider ordering a screen to determine whether a patient's self-report of their prescription drug or substance use is consistent with the patient's actual current clinical state. Psychologists working outside of primary care settings might request this type of test through the primary medical provider.

- *Prescription monitoring systems.* Psychologists can be involved in state prescription monitoring systems, particularly with prescription medications. These are usually available for prescription drugs with high abuse potential, such as controlled opiates and benzodiazepines. Information is stored in a state database with automated alerts that are available when patients go to their local pharmacy. This can provide detailed information about how many different doctors and prescriptions an individual patient may have.

MS. B'S SUD ASSESSMENT SUMMARY

Ms. B exhibits a maladaptive pattern of use stretching over many decades. Her symptoms include tolerance, failed attempts to cut down, spending excessive time and money on alcohol, and ongoing social and occupational impairment. She meets DSM–5 criteria for alcohol dependence. Details of her use were described as follows: In the past, Ms. B would begin drinking at lunchtime with one to two glasses of wine followed by a glass of wine while preparing dinner and two glasses of wine with dinner. Since her hospital stay, she doesn't start drinking until the late afternoon, but she still consumes three to four glasses per day. Alcohol helps her relax and allows her to "forget" her depression. She engages in few activities and is socially isolated. She has conflicts with her daughter, who wants to move Ms. B to an assisted-living facility. Although she would like to think that she can stop drinking on her own, Ms. B recognizes that she needs help and is hoping that her provider may be able to offer this to her. She is somewhat ashamed about her drinking and may not bring it up unless asked directly. Ms. B has suffered from a depressed mood for a number of years that started after her husband died. She has never taken medications for depression because she doesn't think that her depression is that bad. She generally has avoided seeking medical care, as she does not feel comfortable with doctors. She has occasionally visited the acute care clinic for respiratory infections, but does not have a primary care physician whom she has seen on a regular basis. Other than her recent GI incident, she has no comorbid medical conditions. This most recent hospitalization was a wake-up call for her. The doctors told her that the GI bleed was most likely related to her alcohol use and she recognizes that she needs to take better care of herself and get some help with her alcohol dependence. She has never been in a treatment program before but has tried to quit "cold turkey" a number of times without success. She is uncomfortable with the public nature of 12-step programs and wants this to be resolved "quietly and with dignity." No collateral sources of information were used.

Referral to Treatment

During the assessment process, the mental health provider can use strategies to promote patient motivation to change and/or increase the probability of accepting a referral to specialty treatment. A discussion of past quit attempts (and possible withdrawal symptoms), experiences with past treatment programs, and expectations for future treatment programs may provide opportunities to correct misinformation and offer reassurance. Reviewing the pros and cons of use may also serve as an important motivational enhancement tool. A discussion of social and family circumstance could highlight untapped resources or provide additional motivation to get help regarding relationship conflicts or social isolation. In short, although the screening and assessment phase is not technically a "brief intervention" or treatment, assessment may begin to prepare the patient to continue with this important work either with the assessment provider or with another provider delivering specialty care. Below we provide a therapy transcript of the closing exchange with Ms. B—now fully screened, assessed, and ready to accept a specialty referral for alcohol dependence.

Ms. B: Increasing Motivation for Treatment During the Clinical Assessment

Therapist: What worries you most about your drinking?

Ms. B: Well, I wasn't really that *worried* about it until this recent hospital incident. I think it's clear now that I'm drinking too much.

Therapist: That must have been really scary for you.

Ms. B: Yeah. It made me realize too that I'm all alone. My husband passed away and I've lost touch with my daughter and my friends.

Therapist: Lost touch?

Ms. B: Yeah. They say I drink too much . . . I guess we're back to my drinking.

Therapist: Have you tried to cut down or quit?

Ms. B: Oh, yeah. Usually after a fight with my daughter or maybe if I get a bad hangover. Usually I'm all gung-ho at 9 am but by 5 pm I have a glass of wine in my hand. I guess you can't teach an old dog new tricks.

Therapist: It's a really difficult thing to do on your own. Have you ever been in treatment before or seen a therapist?

Ms. B: No. That just seems so extreme.

Therapist: Well, as you know, it's a pretty tough problem to beat without help and it seems like you've suffered enough already.

Ms. B: Well, I'm just not sure.

Therapist: What do you imagine it would be like if you were to go to an alcohol treatment program?

Ms. B: Well, I've seen picture shows where they are in groups and where they show tough love and all that. I don't want to be locked away or anything.

Therapist: OK. Well, it doesn't have to be a residential treatment program. You could live at home and still be around the things that give you comfort. We would want to make sure you are medically monitored just in case you have any withdrawal symptoms. The treatment program might have groups but you could also try it one on one. I know of some excellent programs that specialize in helping older adults.

Ms. B: I think I'd like it to be private.

Therapist: OK, that's fair. As you know, though, this has affected your family and friends, so they might appreciate being told about it and maybe included in your recovery at some point down the road. Is there anything else that worries you about going to treatment?

Ms. B: Well, just the cost, I guess. I'm on a fixed income. Will Medicare cover this?

Therapist: That's a good question. Fortunately, we live in a city with some good treatment options that are fully covered by Medicare. Could we talk about some treatment options for you?

Ms. B: Sure. I'd like to see what's out there.

CONSIDERATIONS FOR CULTURE, DISABILITY, AND COGNITIVE IMPAIRMENT

There is limited information on cultural competence for SBIRT in older substance users. *Culture* can include elements such as race/ethnicity, gender, or socioeconomic status and is generally understood as those factors that may contribute to the development of particular attitudes, beliefs, and values. The limited research on the cultural translation and effectiveness of SBIRT does suggest that protocols developed in the US have been successful in other cultures, such as Poland (Cherpitel, Bernstein, Bernstein, Moskalewicz, & Swiatkiewicz, 2009). SBIRT has also been successfully applied in high-risk, diverse populations, such as Native American pregnant women (Montag, Clapp, Calac, Gorman, & Chambers, 2012).

Important demographic patterns found for SUD in older persons warrant additional consideration. It is expected that by the year 2020, approximately 1.5% of the 73,645 persons ages 50 years and older will meet criteria for an SUD (Han, Gfroerer, Colliver, & Penne, 2009). Demographically, it is projected that a large majority (78.9%) of these will be White (Han et al., 2009). Male older adults will be 2.3 times more likely than their female counterparts to have a past-year SUD, those with fewer than 12 years of education will be about 1.5 times more likely to have a past-year SUD than those with more education, and those who initiated illicit drug use by age 16 will be 4.0 times more likely to have a past-year SUD (Han et al., 2009).

Older patients may be less comfortable with discussions surrounding the acceptability of SBIRT tasks and substance-related discussions due to more traditional or conventional views about substance use (Broyles et al., 2012). Ethnic diversity and prior experiences with prejudice or discrimination may affect accurate assessment during SBIRT. Broyles and colleagues (2012) found that most ethnic minority patients were less accepting of SBIRT techniques. Dobscha, Dickinson, Lasarev, and Lee (2009) reported that in the VA, ethnic minority patients have received more substance-related advice and counseling than their White counterparts, possibly due to racial stereotypes and prejudices. Therefore, as with all therapeutic techniques but especially SBIRT, clinicians are encouraged to foster a conscientiousness and self-reflective awareness of one's own cultural values and biases. This may be especially important when working with ethnic minority clients during the assessment component of SBIRT.

Although limited research has focused specifically on SBIRT for older populations with disability and cognitive impairment, there has been widespread dissemination of SBIRT into emergency departments (Bernstein & D'Onofrio, 2013; Bernstein et al., 2009; Cunningham et al., 2009) where in the United States at least 15% of patients are 65 years or older (Strange, Chen, & Sanders, 1992). SBIRT has also been adopted in primary care settings (Marshall et al., 2012) where older adults often arrive with a complex array of health problems and cognitive impairments.

Disability can serve as both cause and effect of substance use, and cognitive impairment is a common consequence of chronic alcohol or drug use (e.g., Korsakoff's syndrome, Wernicke's encephalopathy). In general, disability is more frequent as one ages, which further contributes to chronic stress. Some cope with the increased stress by using alcohol and drugs. Among the disabled population, the consequences of use are more worrisome, as they may be more severe. For example, those with impaired balance are more likely to fall when intoxicated, resulting in more injuries and impairments. In other cases, SUD may be the primary cause of disability. For this reason, ongoing, careful assessment in the functional and cognitive domains (see the Functional Impairment and Psychosocial/Behavioral Assessment sections in this chapter) is vital to SBIRT with older persons.

Especially with cognitive disability, it is important to examine neurological changes and changes in neuropsychological testing results. SUD can be a major cause of cognitive impairment (e.g., Korsakoff's) and can worsen preexisting cognitive impairment and/or cognitive impairment due to other causes (e.g., Alzheimer's). Continued collaboration with an interdisciplinary team and immediate referrals to the appropriate specialists when problems fall beyond the scope of the clinician's expertise is the best way to address the needs of this population.

CONCLUSION

SBIRT is an effective strategy to recognize and prioritize the clinical and social sequelae of SUD in older persons. However, it is not a foolproof solution. In the general population, there is a 40% to 60% relapse rate for patients treated for alcohol or drug dependence within a year following discharge (McLellan, Lewis, O'Brien, & Kleber, 2000). Nevertheless, those who are connected to treatment generally have more favorable outcomes than those who are not in treatment (McLellan et al., 2000). Therefore, especially with older persons, it may be helpful to view SUD as a condition that will wax and wane but one that does respond to treatment. This chapter followed the case of Ms. B and the application of effective strategies to help identify, address, and guide her toward a reduction in her drinking. Clinical resources were provided that might provide further guidance and assistance for clinicians working with SUD in older persons.

REFERENCES

Adams, W. L., Magruder-Habib, K., Trued, S., & Broome, H. L. (1992). Alcohol abuse in elderly emergency department patients. *Journal of the American Geriatrics Society, 40,* 1236–1240.

American Psychiatric Association. (1994). *Diagnostic and statistical manual of mental disorders* (4th ed.). Washington, DC: Author.

American Psychiatric Association. (2012). *DSM–5 development: Substance use and addictive disorders.* Retrieved from http://www.dsm5.org/ProposedRevision/Pages/SubstanceUseandAddictiveDisorders.aspx

American Psychiatric Association. (2013). *Diagnostic and statistical manual of mental disorders* (5th ed.). Washington, DC: Author.

Atkinson, R. M., Tolson, R. L., & Turner, J. A. (1990). Late versus early onset problem drinking in older men. *Alcoholism: Clinical and Experimental Research, 14,* 574–579. doi:10.1111/j.1530-0277.1990.tb01203.x

Babor, T. F., Biddle-Higgins, J. C., Saunders, J. B., & Monteiro, M. G. (2001). *AUDIT: The Alcohol Use Disorders Identification Test: Guidelines for use in primary health care.* Geneva, Switzerland: World Health Organization.

Babor, T. F., McRee, B. G., Kassebaum, P. A., Grimaldi, P. L., Ahmed, K., & Bray, J. (2007). Screening, brief intervention and referral to treatment (SBIRT): Toward a public health approach to the management of substance abuse. *Substance Abuse, 28,* 7–30. doi:10.1300/J465v28n03_03

Bernstein, E., Topp, D., Shaw, E., Girard, C., Pressman, K., Woolcock, E., & Bernstein, J. (2009). A preliminary report of knowledge translation: Lessons from taking screening and brief intervention techniques from the research setting into regional systems of care. *Academic Emergency Medicine, 16,* 1225–1233. doi:10.1111/j.1553-2712.2009.00516.x

Bernstein, S. L., & D'Onofrio, G. (2013). A promising approach for emergency departments to care for patients with substance use and behavioral disorders. *Health Affairs, 32,* 2122–2128. doi:10.1377/hlthaff.2013.0664

Blazer, D. G., & Wu, L. T. (2009). The epidemiology of substance use and disorders among middle aged and elderly community adults: National survey on drug use and health. *The American Journal of Geriatric Psychiatry, 17,* 237–245. doi:10.1097/JGP.0b013e318190b8ef

Blow, F. C. (1998). *Substance abuse by older adults treatment improvement protocol (TIP).* Rockville, MD: Substance Abuse and Mental Health Services Administration, Office of Applied Studies.

Brown, R. L., Leonard, T., Saunders, L. A., & Papasouliotis, O. (2001). A two-item conjoint screen for alcohol and other drug problems. *The Journal of the American Board of Family Practice, 14,* 95–106.

Broyles, L. M., Rosenberger, E., Hanusa, B. H., Kraemer, K. L., & Gordon, A. J. (2012). Hospitalized patients' acceptability of nurse-delivered screening, brief intervention, and referral to treatment. *Alcoholism: Clinical and Experimental Research, 36,* 725–731. doi:10.1111/j.1530-0277.2011.01651.x

Butler, S. F., Budman, S. H., Fernandez, K., & Jamison, R. N. (2004). Validation of a screener and opioid assessment measure for patients with chronic pain. *Pain, 112,* 65–75. doi:10.1016/j.pain.2004.07.026

Butler, S. F., Fernandez, K., Benoit, C., Budman, S. H., & Jamison, R. N. (2008). Validation of the revised Screener and Opioid Assessment for Patients with Pain (SOAPP-R). *The Journal of Pain, 9,* 360–372. doi:10.1016/j.jpain.2007.11.014

Cherpitel, C. J., Bernstein, E., Bernstein, J., Moskalewicz, J., & Swiatkiewicz, G. (2009). Screening, brief intervention and referral to treatment (SBIRT) in a Polish emergency room: Challenges in cultural translation of SBIRT. *Journal of Addictions Nursing, 20,* 127–131. doi:10.1080/10884600903047618

Chou, R., Fanciullo, G. J., Fine, P. G., Adler, J. A., Ballantyne, J. C., Davies, P., . . . Miaskowsk, C. (2009). American Pain Society-American Academy of Pain Medicine Opioids Guidelines Panel. (2009). Clinical guidelines for the use of chronic opioid therapy in chronic noncancer pain. *The Journal of Pain, 10,* 113–130. doi:10.1016/j.jpain.2008.10.008

Colliver, J. D., Compton, W. M., Gfroerer, J. C., & Condon, T. (2006). Projecting drug use among aging baby boomers in 2020. *Annals of Epidemiology, 16,* 257–265. doi:10.1016/j.annepidem.2005.08.003

Cook, B. L., Winokur, G., Garvey, M. J., & Beach, V. (1991). Depression and previous alcoholism in the elderly. *The British Journal of Psychiatry, 158,* 72–75. doi:10.1192/bjp.158.1.72

Cunningham, R. M., Bernstein, S. L., Walton, M., Broderick, K., Vaca, F. E., Woolard, R., . . . D'Onofrio, G. (2009). Alcohol, tobacco, and other drugs: Future directions for screening and intervention in the emergency department. *Academic Emergency Medicine, 16,* 1078–1088. doi:10.1111/j.1553-2712.2009.00552.x

Davis, L., Uezato, A., Newell, J. M., & Frazier, E. (2008). Major depression and comorbid substance use disorders. *Current Opinion in Psychiatry, 21,* 14–18. doi:10.1097/YCO.0b013e3282f32408

Dobscha, S. K., Dickinson, K. C., Lasarev, M. R., & Lee, E. S. (2009). Associations between race and ethnicity and receipt of advice about alcohol use in the

Department of Veterans Affairs. *Psychiatric Services, 60,* 663–670. doi:10.1176/appi.ps.60.5.663

Dunn, K. M., Saunders, K. W., Rutter, C. M., Banta-Green, C. J., Merrill, J. O., Sullivan, M. D., . . . Von Korff, M. (2010). Opioid prescriptions for chronic pain and overdose: A cohort study. *Annals of Internal Medicine, 152,* 85–92. doi:10.7326/0003-4819-152-2-201001190-00006

Ewing, J. A. (1984). Detecting alcoholism. The CAGE questionnaire. *JAMA, 252,* 1905–1907. doi:10.1001/jama.1984.03350140051025

Fahmy, V., Hatch, S. L., Hotopf, M., & Stewart, R. (2012). Prevalences of illicit drug use in people aged 50 years and over from two surveys. *Age and Ageing.* Advance online publication. Retrieved from http://ageing.oxfordjournals.org/content/early/2012/03/16/ageing.afs020.long

Fiore, M. C., Jaen, C. R., Baker, T. B., Bailey, W. C., Benowitz, N. L., Curry, S. J., . . . Wewers, M. E. (2008). *Treating tobacco use and dependence: 2008 update.* Washington, DC: U.S. Department of Health and Human Services. Retrieved from http://www.ahrq.gov/professionals/clinicians-providers/guidelines recommendations/tobacco/clinicians/update/treating_tobacco_use08.pdf

Fleming, M. F., Davis, J., & Passik, S. D. (2008). Reported lifetime aberrant drug-taking behaviors are predictive of current substance use and mental health problems in primary care patients. *Pain Medicine, 9,* 1098–1106. doi:10.1111/j.1526-4637.2008.00491.x

Friedmann, P. D., McCullough, D., Chin, M. H., & Saitz, R. (2000). Screening and intervention for alcohol problems. A national survey of primary care physicians and psychiatrists. *Journal of General Internal Medicine, 15,* 84–91. doi:10.1046/j.1525-1497.2000.03379.x

Gavin, D. R., Ross, H. E., & Skinner, H. A. (1989). Diagnostic validity of the drug abuse screening test in the assessment of *DSM–III* drug disorders. *British Journal of Addiction, 84,* 301–307. doi:10.1111/j.1360-0443.1989.tb03463.x

Gfroerer, J. C., & Epstein, J. F. (1999). Marijuana initiates and their impact on future drug abuse treatment need. *Drug and Alcohol Dependence, 54,* 229–237. doi:10.1016/S0376-8716(98)00167-7

Gfroerer, J. C., Penne, M., Pemberton, M., & Folsom, R. (2003). Substance abuse treatment need among older adults in 2020: The impact of the aging baby-boom cohort. *Drug and Alcohol Dependence, 69,* 127–135. doi:10.1016/S0376-8716(02)00307-1

Han, B., Gfroerer, J. C., Colliver, J. D., & Penne, M. C. (2009). Substance use disorder among older adults in the United States in 2020. *Addiction, 104,* 88–96. doi:10.1111/j.1360-0443.2008.02411.x

Huang, B., Dawson, D. A., Stinson, F. S., Hasin, D. S., Ruan, W. J., Saha, T. D., . . . Grant, B. F. (2006). Prevalence, correlates, and comorbidity of non-medical prescription drug use and drug use disorders in the United States: Results for the National Epidemiologic Survey on Alcohol and Related Conditions. *Journal of Clinical Psychiatry, 67,* 1062–1073. doi:10.4088/JCP.v67n0708

Katz, S., Ford, A. B., Moskowitz, R. W., Jackson, B. A., & Jaffe, M. W. (1963). Studies of illness in the aged: The index of ADL: a standardized measure of biological and psychosocial function. *JAMA, 185*, 914–919. doi:10.1001/jama.1963.03060120024016

Kendell, R., & Jablensky, A. (2003). Distinguishing between the validity and utility of psychiatric diagnoses. *The American Journal of Psychiatry, 160*, 4–12. doi:10.1176/appi.ajp.160.1.4

Kohlman-Thomson, L. (1992). *Kohlman evaluation of living skills* (3rd ed.). Bethesda, MD: American Occupational Therapy Association.

Kypri, K., Langley, J. D., Saunders, J. B., Cashell-Smith, M. L., & Herbison, P. (2008). Randomized controlled trial of web-based alcohol screening and brief intervention in primary care. *Archives of Internal Medicine, 168*, 530–536. doi:10.1001/archinternmed.2007.109

Lee, J. D., Delbanco, B., Wu, E., & Gourevitch, M. N. (2011). Substance use prevalence and screening instrument comparisons in urban primary care. *Substance Abuse, 32*, 128–134. doi:10.1080/08897077.2011.562732

Lee, Y., Back, J. H., Kim, J., Kim, S. H., Na, D. L., Cheong, H. K., . . . Kim, Y. G. (2010). Systematic review of health behavioral risks and cognitive health in older adults. *International Psychogeriatrics, 22*, 174–187. doi:10.1017/S1041610209991189

Lemke, S., & Moos, R.H. (2003). Treatment and outcomes of older patients with alcohol use disorders in community residential programs. *Journal of Studies in Alcohol, 64*, 219–226.

Liebschutz, J. M., & Alford, D. P. (2011). Safe opioid prescribing: A long way to go. *Journal of General Internal Medicine, 26*, 951–952. doi:10.1007/s11606-011-1797-3

Lin, J. C., Karno, M. P., Grella, C. E., Warda, U., Liao, D. H., Hu, P., & Moore, A. A. (2011). Alcohol, tobacco, and non-medical drug use disorders in U.S. adults aged 65 and older: Data from the 2001–2002 National Epidemiologic Survey of Alcohol and Related Conditions. *The American Journal of Geriatric Psychiatry, 19*, 292–299. doi:10.1097/JGP.0b013e3181e898b4

Loeb, P. A. (1996). *Independent Living Scales*. San Antonio, TX: The Psychological Corporation.

Maciosek, M. V., Coffield, A. B., Edwards, N. M., Flottemesch, T. J., Goodman, M. J., & Solberg, L. I. (2006). Priorities among effective clinical preventive services: Results of a systematic review and analysis. *American Journal of Preventive Medicine, 31*, 52–61. doi:10.1016/j.amepre.2006.03.012

Madras, B. K., Compton, W. M., Avula, D., Stegbauer, T., Stein, J. B., & Clark, H. W. (2009). Screening, brief interventions, referral to treatment (SBIRT) for illicit drug and alcohol use at multiple healthcare sites: Comparison at intake and 6 months later. *Drug and Alcohol Dependence, 99*, 280–295. doi:10.1016/j.drugalcdep.2008.08.003

Marshall, V. J., McLaurin-Jones, T. L., Kalu, N., Kwagyan, J., Scott, D. M., Cain, G . . . Taylor, R. E. (2012). Screening, brief intervention, and referral to treatment:

Public health training for primary care. *American Journal of Public Health, 102,* e30–e36. doi:10.2105/AJPH.2012.300802

McLellan, A. T., Lewis, D. C., O'Brien, C. P., & Kleber, H. D. (2000). Drug dependence, a chronic medical illness: implications for treatment, insurance, and outcomes evaluation. *JAMA, 284,* 1689–1695.

Meltzer, E. C., Rybin, D., Saitz, R., Samet, J. H., Schwartz, S. L., Butler, S. F., & Liebschutz, J. M. (2011). Identifying prescription opioid use disorder in primary care: Diagnostic characteristics of the Current Opioid Misuse Measure (COMM). *Pain, 152,* 397–402. doi:10.1016/j.pain.2010.11.006

Montag, A., Clapp, J. D., Calac, D., Gorman, J., & Chambers, C. (2012). A review of evidence-based approaches for reduction of alcohol consumption in Native women who are pregnant or of reproductive age. *The American Journal of Drug and Alcohol Abuse, 38,* 436–443. doi:10.3109/00952990.2012.694521

Moos, R. H., Brennan, P. L., Schutte, K. K., & Moos, B. S. (2004). High-risk alcohol consumption and late-life alcohol use problems. *American Journal of Public Health, 94,* 1985–1991. doi:10.2105/AJPH.94.11.1985

Okie, S. (2010). A flood of opioids, a rising tide of deaths. *The New England Journal of Medicine, 363,* 1981–1985. doi:10.1056/NEJMp1011512

Organization of Economic Cooperation and Development. (2011). Old-age income poverty. In *Pensions at a Glance, 2011: Retirement-income systems in OECD and G20 countries.* Paris, France: OECD.

Oslin, D. W., Pettinati, H., & Volpicelli, J. R. (2002). Alcoholism treatment adherence: Older age predicts better adherence and drinking outcomes. *The American Journal of Geriatric Psychiatry, 10,* 740–747. doi:10.1097/00019442-200211000-00013

Passik, S. D., & Kirsh, K. L. (2004). Assessing aberrant drug-taking behaviors in the patient with chronic pain. *Current Pain and Headache Reports, 8,* 289–294. doi:10.1007/s11916-004-0010-3

Passik, S. D., & Kirsh, K. L. (2008). The interface between pain and drug abuse and the evolution of strategies to optimize pain management while minimizing drug abuse. *Experimental and Clinical Psychopharmacology, 16,* 400–404. doi:10.1037/a0013634

Pringle, K. E., Ahem, F. M., Heller, D. A., Gold, C. H., & Brown, T. V. (2005). Potential for alcohol and prescription drug interactions in older people. *Journal of the American Geriatrics Society, 53,* 1930. doi:10.1111/j.1532–5415.2005.00474.x

Rigler, S. K. (2000). Alcoholism in the elderly. *American Family Physician, 61,* 1710–1716.

Satre, D. D., Sterling, S. A., Mackin, R. S., & Weisner, C. (2011). Patterns of alcohol and drug use among depressed older adults seeking outpatient psychiatric services. *The American Journal of Geriatric Psychiatry, 19,* 695–703. doi:10.1097/JGP.0b013e3181f17f0a

Saunders, J. B., Aasland, O. G., Babor, T. F., de la Fuente, J. R., & Grant, M. (1993). Development of the Alcohol Use Disorders Identification Test (AUDIT):

WHO Collaborative Project on Early Detection of Persons with Harmful Alcohol Consumption—II. *Addiction, 88,* 791–804. doi:10.1111/j.1360-0443.1993.tb02093.x

Saunders, P. A., Copeland, J. R., Dewey, M. E., Davidson, I. A., McWilliam, C., Sharma, V., & Sullivan, C. (1991). Heavy drinking as a risk factor for depression and dementia in elderly men: Findings from the Liverpool longitudinal community study. *The British Journal of Psychiatry, 159,* 213–216. doi:10.1192/bjp.159.2.213

Schonfeld, L., & Dupree, L.W. (1991). Antecedents of drinking for early- and late-onset elderly alcohol abusers. *Journal of Studies on Alcohol, 52,* 587–592.

Schonfeld, L., King-Kallimanis, B. L., Duchene, D. M., Etheridge, R. L., Herrera, J. R., Barry, K. L., & Lynn, N. (2010). Screening and brief intervention for substance misuse among older adults: The Florida BRITE project. *American Journal of Public Health, 100,* 108–114. doi:10.2105/AJPH.2008.149534

Simoni-Wastila, L., & Yang, H. K. (2006). Psychoactive drug abuse in older adults. *American Journal of Geriatric Pharmacotherapy, 4,* 380–394. doi:10.1016/j.amjopharm.2006.10.002

Simoni-Wastila, L., Zuckerman, I. H., Singhal, P. K., Briesacher, B., & Hsu, V. D. (2006). National estimates of exposure to prescription drugs with addiction potential in community-dwelling elders. *Substance Abuse, 26,* 33–42. doi:10.1300/J465v26n01_04

Skinner, H. A. (1982). The drug abuse screening test. *Addictive Behaviors, 7,* 363–371.

Smith, P. C., Schmidt, S. M., Allensworth-Davies, D., & Saitz, R. (2010). A single-question screening test for drug use in primary care. *Archives of Internal Medicine, 170,* 1155–1160. doi:10.1001/archinternmed.2010.140

Solberg, L. I., Maciosek, M. V., & Edwards, N. M. (2008). Primary care intervention to reduce alcohol misuse: Ranking its health impact and cost effectiveness. *American Journal of Preventive Medicine, 34,* 143–152. doi:10.1016/j.amepre.2007.09.035

Strange, G. R., Chen, E. H., & Sanders, A. B. (1992). Use of emergency departments by elderly patients: Projections from a multicenter database. *Annals of Emergency Medicine, 21,* 819–824. doi:10.1016/S0196-0644(05)81028-5

Substance Abuse and Mental Health Services Administration. (1998). *Substance abuse among older adults. Treatment Improvement Protocol (TIP), Series No. 26.* Rockville, MD: Center for Substance Abuse Treatment.

Substance Abuse and Mental Health Services Administration. (2005). *The National Survey on Drug Use and Health: Substance use among older adults: 2002 and 2003 Update.* Retrieved from http://www.oas.samhsa.gov/2k5/olderadults/olderadults.htm

Substance Abuse and Mental Health Services Administration. (2011). *Illicit drug use among older adults.* Retrieved from http://www.samhsa.gov/data/2k11/WEB_SR_013/WEB_SR_013.htm

Substance Abuse and Mental Health Services Administration. (2012). *Office of Applied Studies. Substance abuse treatment admissions involving abuse of pain relievers: 1998–2008.* Retrieved from http://oas.samhsa.gov/2k10/230/230PainRelvr2k10.cfm

United States Preventive Services Task Force. (2012). *Screening and behavioral counseling interventions in primary care to reduce alcohol misuse.* Retrieved from http://www.uspreventiveservicestaskforce.org/uspstf/uspsdrin.htm

Vestal, R. E., McGuire, E. A., Tobin, J. D., Andres, R., Norris, A. H., & Mezey, E. (1977). Aging and ethanol metabolism. *Clinical Pharmacology and Therapeutics, 21*, 343–354.

Watson, I. D., Berthold, R., Hammett-Stabler, C., Nicholes, B., Smith, B., George, S., . . . Goldberger, B. (2006). Drugs and ethanol. In J. H. Nicholds (Ed.), *Laboratory medicine practice guidelines: Evidence-based practice for point-of-care testing* (pp. 63–75). Washington, DC: National Academy of Clinical Biochemistry.

World Health Organization ASSIST Working Group. (2002). The Alcohol, Smoking and Substance Involvement Screening Test (ASSIST): Development, reliability and feasibility. *Addiction, 97*, 1183–1194.

World Health Organization Suicide Prevention (SUPRE). (2012). *Suicide prevention (SUPRE).* Retrieved from http://www.who.int/mental_health/prevention/suicide/suicideprevent/en/

Wu, L. T., & Blazer, D. G. (2011). Illicit and nonmedical drug use among older adults: A review. *Journal of Aging and Health, 23*, 481–504. doi:10.1177/0898264310386224

Yudko, E., Lozhkina, O., & Fouts, A. (2007). A comprehensive review of the psychometric properties of the Drug Abuse Screening Test. *Journal of Substance Abuse Treatment, 32*, 189–198. doi:10.1016/j.jsat.2006.08.002

9

RELAPSE PREVENTION TREATMENT FOR SUBSTANCE ABUSE DISORDERS IN OLDER ADULTS

LAWRENCE SCHONFELD AND NICOLE S. MacFARLAND

Research suggests that the use of substances among older adults might double or even triple by 2020, based on national household surveys assessing lifetime use of marijuana, illicit drug use, and the nonmedical use of prescription medications among the baby boom population (Blazer & Wu, 2009; Colliver, Compton, Gfroerer, & Condon, 2006). Given the rapid aging of the U.S. population, changes in delivery of services as the result of implementation of the Affordable Health Care for America Act (H. R. 3962) and enhanced access to behavioral health services, the increasing numbers of older adults requiring substance abuse treatment might overwhelm existing resources.

In this chapter, we describe the challenges of identifying and treating older adults with substance use disorders (SUDs). We apply the relapse prevention (RP) model to the case example of "Mr. M," an older adult with problems related to abuse of alcohol and prescription medications. The Substance Abuse and Mental Health Services Administration's (SAMHSA's) National

http://dx.doi.org/10.1037/14524-010
Treatment of Late-Life Depression, Anxiety, Trauma, and Substance Abuse, P. A. Areán (Editor)

Registry of Evidence-based Programs and Practices (NREPP; SAMHSA, 2014) lists relapse prevention therapy (RPT) among its highly rated practices. RPT, first implemented in 1977, has been tested across numerous studies, categories of substances, and varied populations. Using this model, and the methodologies identified in a SAMHSA manual specific to relapse prevention for older adults, we describe how treatment providers can work with clients to effectively identify each person's high-risk situation and teach him or her the skills necessary to avoid lapses and prevent relapses.

We begin our discussion with the criteria used to identify and diagnose SUDs. Next, we address these issues specific to an older population. We then discuss the strategies included within an age-specific RP approach, and, last, we apply these strategies to a case example.

IDENTIFICATION AND DIAGNOSTIC CRITERIA

The first challenge in addressing SUDs is to identify those who meet diagnostic criteria and engage them in some form of intervention or treatment, with older adults presenting several additional challenges to standard criteria. Among the general population, individuals meeting diagnostic criteria for one or more SUDs can be admitted to formal substance abuse treatment programs. Briefly summarized, the previous *Diagnostic and Statistical Manual of Mental Disorders* (DSM; fourth edition, text revision; American Psychiatric Association, 2000) diagnostic criteria for substance abuse utilized the dichotomy of abuse and dependence. A *substance abuse disorder* refers to a pattern of substance use leading to significant impairment or distress in the past 12 months, with endorsement of at least one of four criteria: (1) failure to fulfill major role obligations at work, school, home; (2) frequent use of substances in situations in which it is physically hazardous; (3) frequent legal problems; and (4) continued use despite having persistent or recurrent social or interpersonal problems. *Substance use dependence* is a "maladaptive pattern of substance use, leading to clinically significant impairment or distress" over a 12-month period. Criteria include three or more of the following criteria: (1) changes in tolerance, (2) withdrawal symptoms, (3) consuming larger amounts or for longer duration, (4) difficulties in cutting down or control, (5) spending a great deal of time trying to obtain the substance, (6) giving up activities or reducing activities because of substance use, or (7) continuing despite knowledge of physical or psychological problems caused or exacerbated by the substance use. Changes in the DSM–5 (American Psychiatric Association, 2013) for SUDs include categorizing them on a continuum of severity rather than the dichotomy of abuse versus dependence, relying less on criteria of physical tolerance and withdrawal symptoms, and forgoing the term *addiction* in favor of *use disorder*. As noted by Compton, Dawson, Goldstein, and Grant (2013), the

> 11 *DSM–5* SUD criteria comprise a new craving criterion plus all the former *DSM–IV* abuse and dependence criteria except substance-related recurrent legal problems. Mild *DSM–5* SUD requires endorsement of 2–3 of these criteria, moderate SUD requires 4–5, and severe SUD requires 6 criteria. (p. 387)

Identification of older adults' problems with alcohol, medications, and illicit drugs may be a challenge when using these criteria. With age-related changes in metabolism, older adults may require consumption of lower quantities of alcohol to achieve the effects experienced when they were younger. Such declines in tolerance contrast young adults' increases in tolerance for alcohol consumption with continued heavy or problematic drinking. A second challenge in identifying SUDs for older adults pertains to the characteristics of medication misuse. Younger adults may be diagnosed with an SUD related to opioids, amphetamines, or other medications that may be obtained illegally and used for recreational or other nonmedical purposes. In contrast, older adults may begin with legitimately prescribed medications for chronic medical problems but may become dependent due to prescribing practices, or they may commit errors in taking their medications due to confusion resulting from handling multiple prescribed medications, memory problems, medication interactions, and other circumstances that do not imply intentional misuse. Furthermore, many medications (e.g., benzodiazepines) are fat soluble, leading to longer half-lives of the active ingredients and greater dependency.

Epidemiological studies based on household surveys and treatment admission data differ with respect to the conclusions one might draw about the need for treatment of substance abuse among the older population. First, definitions of terms such as *older adults* or *elderly* vary greatly within the published literature. State-level and local aging services serve individuals ages 60 and older, state-level behavioral health services may serve 55 and older, and federal programs such as Medicare and Social Security generally serve age 65 and older. These variations affect the target population in need of treatment services. Second, it would appear that the household survey data do not influence admissions since, traditionally, younger adults in their 20s and 30s are more often admitted to formal treatment. A review of the 10-year period 2000–2010 shows that for treatment admissions for alcohol, illicit drugs, and medications, age-group rates of admissions dropped off rapidly beginning around age 50 and irrespective of race/ethnicity or gender (SAMHSA, 2012).

Despite the dropoff in admissions, trends in the household survey data suggest that the baby boom population will have greater needs for treatment. In the older population, as in other age groups, alcohol remains the substance most frequently addressed in substance abuse treatment programs. Over the years, results from the National Survey on Drug Use and Health (NSDUH) have demonstrated the extent to which older individuals use and misuse substances. For example, in the 2002/2003 NSDUH data, for past-month use, 12.2% of those ages 50 and older reported binge alcohol use and 3.2% reported heavy alcohol use; 1.8% reported using an illicit drug in the past month, most frequently marijuana followed by nonmedical use of prescription drugs and cocaine. While a greater proportion of younger than older adults use these substances, trends suggest increasing problems for the baby boom generation. For example, between 2002 and 2010 the rate of illicit drug use more than doubled (from 3.4% to 7.2%) for adults ages 50 to 54 and those ages 55 to 59 (from 1.9% to 4.1%), demonstrating the impact of the baby boom cohort (SAMHSA, 2011).

Older adults are more likely than younger adults to have multiple medical problems, are prescribed more medications (often with difficult regimens), and are more likely to experience age-related sensitivities to the medications. As a result, treatment for medication misuse will involve patient education on medication management and may also involve coordination of care with the prescribing physician to reduce side effects and the risk of patient errors. Physicians play a key role in this process and may be unaware of side effects or the risks involved in prescribing certain medications that have been judged as inappropriate for older adults (ages 65 and older) using the updated Beers Criteria (American Geriatrics Society, 2012). The Beers criteria are used for improving physicians' selection of prescription medications, educating clinicians and patients on proper use, evaluating health outcomes and costs, and most importantly, improving care of older adults by reducing their exposure to "potentially inappropriate medications."

Due to the way medications are prescribed and used, intentional misuse is more frequent in younger than older adults, as shown in the data from the NSDUH for 2002–2004. Older adults had the lowest rate among age groups (1% for ages 60–64, 0.4% for ages 65 and older) of nonmedical use of pain relievers. Prevalence rates for intentional misuse were highest among the emerging adults (19–21 years) for tranquilizers (5.7%), stimulants (4.8%), and methamphetamine (2.0%). Rates for sedative use were low and did not show as strong an association with age as did rates for misuse of other classes of prescription drugs.

The above discussion is presented so that treatment for older adults can be tailored to the characteristics of use of medications. We need to avoid assumptions that all individuals demonstrating overuse or improper use of prescription medications are intentionally doing so for nontherapeutic reasons. Sometimes medication education may be the most appropriate and briefest method of intervening.

IMPLICATIONS OF CULTURE, DISABILITY,
AND COGNITIVE IMPAIRMENT

These issues present additional challenges for the identification and treatment of older adults with SUDs. In this section, we describe how culture, disability, and cognitive impairment are presented in the scientific literature and how they pose challenges for clinicians who treat older adults.

Cultural Issues

Cultural issues encompass not only race and ethnicity but also the age-related biases often associated with addressing older adults' behavioral health. Professional ageism may influence professionals' judgments when identifying problems among older adults. For example, clinicians might judge slurred speech and memory problems as indicating cognitive impairment and might not consider alcohol consumption or adverse medication reactions. Furthermore, indicators typically used to identify substance use in younger and middle-aged adults (e.g., absences from work, driving under the influence, neglect of child care, marital problems) may have little meaning when assessing, for example, a retired, widowed, older adult.

Racial, ethnic, and gender differences in treatment admissions among adults ages 50 and older were reported in SAMHSA's DASIS (Drug and Alcohol Services Information System) Report (2006), which reported that 72% of those categorized as alcohol-only admissions were White, 14% were Black, and 9% were classified as Hispanic. Among admissions to treatment for other substances, the numbers shifted: 45% White, 40% Black, and 12% Hispanic. According to a 2010 NSDUH report (SAMHSA, 2010), American Indians and Alaska Natives ages 50 and older have somewhat lower rates of alcohol use than the national average but slightly higher rates of binge drinking and illicit drug use than the national average.

The data indicate that even though there may be greater illicit drug use among older members of ethnic minorities, they are less likely to be admitted to treatment. This suggests the need to increase culturally appropriate outreach efforts to these underserved groups.

As is typically found in the younger population, older adult men outnumber older adult women in admissions. The results from the NSDUH household surveys also support this predominance of males over females for illicit drug use but similar rates for nonmedical use of prescription medications.

In sum, these data indicate differences based on race, ethnicity, and sex and suggest the need to increase outreach efforts that are sensitive to communities' values, language, and culture. Once individuals are admitted to formal substance abuse treatment, an approach that is tailored to each client's needs should be more culturally appropriate and age-appropriate.

Disability

The U.S. Office of Disability (2014) reported that more than 54 million Americans have physical or mental disabilities, and one estimate is that 4.7 million have co-occurring disability and SUD, with 50% of persons with traumatic brain injuries, spinal cord injuries, or mental illness experiencing an SUD in comparison with 10% of the general population. The report also suggests that people with deafness, arthritis, or multiple sclerosis have at least double the rate of SUDs compared with the general population. However, these estimates typically pertain to the younger population and little research has been conducted on SUDs in disabled older adults. There is no doubt that use of alcohol and drugs is associated with accidents and injuries that can leave a person disabled. Less known are the challenges related to disabled older adults who also have substance abuse problems. One reason is that the term *disability* has many definitions, pathways, and trajectories. Disabilities of hearing and sight may create challenges for understanding skills taught in substance abuse treatment programs, unless special accommodations are offered by the treatment program.

Physical disabilities that prevent the older adult from commuting to a treatment program are a major challenge. Clinicians would need to understand the person's access to the problem substances; for example, the clinician would need to know how a person who is unable to get to treatment can access alcohol or drugs. If transportation is provided by another, who is that person, and can the intervention begin with him or her? Second, can the clinical program work with local aging services to explore the possibility of providing publicly funded, wheelchair/assisted transportation? Clinicians may try alternatives by providing in-home or telephone counseling in such cases.

Cognitive Impairment

There is a substantial body of literature demonstrating the detrimental effects excessive alcohol consumption has in terms of cognitive impairment, but there is almost no information about the relationship between cognitive impairment and long-term use of illicit substances. Clinicians will be challenged to determine whether observed dementia-like symptoms are temporary, perhaps due to effects of substances in the system or to short-term effects from other issues (e.g., transient ischemic attacks), or whether symptoms are irreversible, and then to determine whether either stage is related to risky or abusive drinking. Gupta and Warner (2008) suggested that clinicians use a label of *probable alcohol-related dementia* only after at least 60 days since last exposure to alcohol, significant alcohol use for more than 5 years, and significant alcohol use occurring within 3 years of the symptom onset.

Studies have investigated the effects of abstinence, limited moderate drinking, and excessive alcohol consumption over the long term. Among the most recent was a study by Sabia et al. (2014), who reported the results of a 10 year British longitudinal study involving 5,054 men and 2,099 women. Cognitive tests were repeated three times over the study. Heavier alcohol consumption (30 grams or more per day) was associated with faster decline in all aspects of cognitive function compared with no differences in cognitive decline among abstainers, quitters, and light or moderate male drinkers. For women, they reported weaker evidence of this effect, with lesser levels of 19 grams/day, and only for executive function.

Among the best-known diagnostic categories is Wernicke-Korsakoff syndrome, which is actually two separate syndromes. Wernicke encephalopathy is characterized by an acute/subacute confusional state and is often reversible. In contrast, Korsakoff dementia is associated with thiamine deficiency due to poor nutrition and heavy drinking and is characterized as persistent and irreversible (Alzheimer's Association, 2014). Research indicates rates of 1% to 3% following autopsies, but it is also believed that many more cases are missed in clinical diagnoses.

Treatment programs will need to examine their admission criteria to determine whether a diagnosis of dementia is an exclusionary criterion. In many cases, a person with mild cognitive impairment (MCI), as assessed by standard neuropsychological screens, can benefit from a structured, elder-friendly group treatment environment. Cognitive behavioral interventions can be used with people with MCI but may need to be adjusted so that there is support from the family, spouse, or significant others. As with the disability issue, a clinician would need to determine how the person with MCI is obtaining the substance and whether that access can be modified.

RELAPSE PREVENTION MODEL FOR OLDER ADULTS

The RP model has been applied to older adults in a small number of studies by the first author and colleagues. In general, the need for treatment should be approached such that the level of service matches the level of assessed risk of alcohol or drug problems. SAMHSA's Treatment Improvement Protocol on Substance Abuse Among Older Adults (CSAT, 1998) notes that brief interventions are appropriate for those demonstrating behaviors that place them at moderate risk for problems related to substance use, whereas brief therapies or brief treatments are best suited for moderate to high risk. SAMHSA's SBIRT initiative includes "referral to treatment" when substance use is severe enough to require more extensive treatment. It is this latter category that was appropriate for the case we describe in this chapter. While family history of substance abuse certainly influences the environment and culture in which the person is raised, the RP model focuses on recent antecedent events and consequences for treatment planning rather than long-term history.

As cited in CSAT (1998, 1999) Treatment Improvement Protocols, Figure 9.1 conceptualizes how the level of service matches the level of severity of the substance abuse problem. At the far left side of the figure is the largest group of people: those whose behavior indicates "none to mild" risk and who could benefit from education about substance use rather than formal treatment. Those at "mild to moderate" risk will benefit from one or two brief advice or brief intervention sessions in which a health educator uses motivational interviewing and education to foster changes in their behavior, which is the same approach used in the Florida BRITE (Brief Intervention and Treatment for Elders) Project (Schonfeld et al., 2010). Finally, people who demonstrate "substantial to severe" risk represent a smaller percentage of the

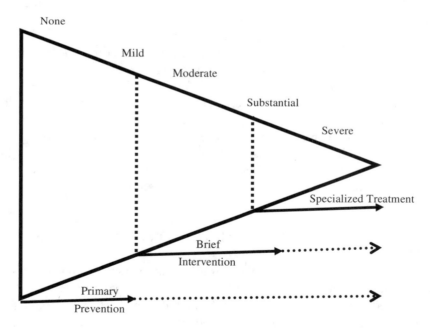

Figure 9.1. Substance abuse severity. From *Broadening the Base of Treatment for Alcohol Problems* (p. 30), by the Institute of Medicine, 1990, Washington, DC: National Academies Press. Copyright 1990 by the National Academy of Sciences. Adapted with permission.

population. They will benefit most from admission to formal treatment that is tailored to their treatment needs. This is the process used within SBIRT.

Age-Specific Treatment

Several studies have suggested that treatment outcomes for older alcohol abusers would be improved in elder-specific group treatment settings versus mixed-age group treatment settings. For example, in one study comparing an elder-specific cohort of veterans in group treatment versus a cohort in mixed-age group treatment (Kofoed, Tolson, Atkinson, Toth, & Turner, 1987), the former resulted in fewer relapses and a longer time between relapses when they occurred. Findings from treatment programs reveal that antecedents or high-risk situations leading to drinking for older adults differ from those for younger adults (Carstensen, Rychtarik, & Prue, 1985; Dupree, Broskowski, & Schonfeld, 1984; Graham, Brett, & Baron, 1997; Schonfeld et al., 2000). Older adults more often use substances because of social isolation and negative mood (primarily depression, loneliness, and boredom). Medical problems are more prevalent for elders and should be addressed in treatment. In contrast, younger adults are more likely to drink or use multiple substances and often in response to peer pressure, socialization, and conflicts with others (Schonfeld, Dupree, & Rohrer, 1995).

As a result, designing treatment approaches for older adults should provide a strategy that determines which skills should be taught in order to prevent relapse should these high-risk situations arise during, or after discharge from, treatment. Furthermore, most of the published research has focused on older adults' drinking problems, while far fewer have addressed other substance use problems, such as use of illicit drugs (i.e., street drugs such as marijuana, crack cocaine, heroin), which appears to be on the rise (Colliver et al., 2006), and also misuse of prescription medications, as in the case of Mr. M.

Assessment as a Treatment-Planning Tool

Assessment instruments that rely on indicators or symptoms common among younger adults often are not pertinent to the treatment needs of older adults. Many older problem drinkers are widowed or divorced, retired, do not drive, and often drink at home and alone (Dupree et al., 1984; Schonfeld et al., 2000). Therefore, the probability that their drinking will be detected by significant others is reduced. Other indicators, such as in-home assessments conducted by an aging services case manager, may be useful in identifying "hidden abusers." In addition, physical symptoms such as complaints about sleeping habits, memory problems, liver function abnormalities, and slurred speech may be mistakenly viewed as age-related illnesses when alcohol or medication misuse could be the culprit.

Relapse Prevention Therapy: Case Example

Mr. M's case is an example of this category given his years of engaging in alcohol abuse, doctor shopping, and seeking pain medications. We selected a case example based, in part, on a patient admitted to Senior Hope Counseling in Albany, New York. Senior Hope was founded in 2002 and is an outpatient, nonintensive, not-for-profit addictions clinic for people ages 50 and older. It offers age-specific groups designed to help older adults. Interdisciplinary treatment teams of medical and counseling staff provide educational approaches, support groups, medication education, and stress management techniques. Using the history and presenting problems identified at admission, we describe how the RP model would be implemented.

Initial Evaluation

Mr. M was a 65-year-old, divorced, Caucasian male referred to Senior Hope in 2008 for an evaluation by his primary care physician due to concerns around possible abuse of prescription medication. He was a college-educated retired insurance agent.

The initial evaluation revealed a history of drug-seeking behavior and alcoholism, as well as one recent and three previous offenses of driving while intoxicated (DWI) over the previous 10 years. Mr. M was very concerned that his most recent DWI, which resulted in an injury to himself, would lead to possible incarceration and loss of his driver's license. Furthermore, injuries from several motorcycle accidents over the years have led to chronic, debilitating pain in his left shoulder and back. The most recent accident exacerbated the problems with his left shoulder, resulting in the need for surgery. Mr. M reported that his physician prescribed pain medication but that the medication was not working. As a result, he sought other physicians to obtain additional pain medication.

Medical History

Mr. M's medical history indicates high cholesterol, nerve damage to his left shoulder, and ongoing chronic pain in his shoulder and back. He has had multiple operations to alleviate the pain in his shoulder. He has also been taking medication prescribed by his primary care physician for the shoulder pain, as well as receiving steroid injections to alleviate the back pain over the years.

Substance Use Diagnoses

Mr. M began using alcohol at age 22 and had been consuming greater amounts of alcohol over the past several years. He last used alcohol 1 week prior to his evaluation. He smoked a pack of cigarettes per day. He met criteria for alcohol dependence as well as nicotine dependence during intake. His prescribed pain medications included a fentanyl patch, Tylenol with codeine, and oxycodone to help manage his shoulder and back pain. He was "doctor shopping" and medication seeking due to increased tolerance of his medications and his chronic pain.

Family History

Mr. M was raised in upstate New York. He reported that his mother struggled with alcoholism with mood fluctuations. His sister and brother both abused alcohol as well. His father used cocaine to cope with the stress of working two jobs. The patient had a history of struggling in relationships with dependent women and had three marriages that resulted in divorce. His two children from his last marriage are currently under the age of 18.

As noted earlier, assessments that rely on indicators or symptoms common among younger substance abusers often are not pertinent to the treatment needs of older adults. Therefore, the assessment process used in the RP model does not use a one-size-fits-all approach; instead, the individualized, structured interview is used to reveal how recent substance use behavior has typically occurred. The information is key to planning which skills will need to be taught and how treatment providers can measure success. The assessment process within the RP model has three stages, as discussed next using Mr. M's case.

Stage 1: Functional Analysis of Substance Use Behavior

A functional analysis of drinking behavior or use of other substances is different from checklists or interview-style assessments that rely on the presence or absence of symptoms. In the RP model for older adults (CSAT, 2005), a structured interview is used to identify antecedents that precede substance use on a typical day of use and to identify both positive and negative consequences of using that substance. This creates the A-B-C (antecedent-behavior-consequences) chain that permits therapist and client to examine the information and take the mystery out of substance use behavior. The goals are to identify each person's high-risk situations for consuming alcohol or illicit drugs so that treatment plans can be individualized.

Early work in developing an RP model for older adults was conducted in Florida during the late 1970s and early 1980s in the Gerontology Alcohol

Project (Dupree et al., 1984) and subsequent versions/adaptations of that program. In the Gerontology Alcohol Project, an elder-appropriate modification of Marlatt's (1976) Drinking Profile was developed and implemented as a treatment planning tool. A later, modified version known as the Substance Abuse Profile for the Elderly (SAPE) was soon developed and published in the CSAT RP curriculum manual (CSAT, 2005).

Applying the approach to Mr. M's drinking behavior, the interview identified specific components of his substance use behavior chain. While the SAPE also includes information about drinking history over the life span, the most recent and typical behavior is the focus for treatment planning. After completing the interview, the counselor and Mr. M reviewed the antecedents identified in terms of situations, thoughts, feelings, cues, and urges that precede the first use of the preferred substance on a typical day of use. They also identified short-term or immediate positive consequences that served to reinforce the behavior as well as short-term and longer term negative consequences that typically followed that first drink.

Using this method, the counselor records a client's responses and provides him or her a transcribed copy for reference in treatment groups. Figure 9.2 illustrates the A-B-Cs substance use behavior chain. The top row illustrates the basic A-B-C chain. The second row describes the general components of each that are identified through the questions on the SAPE. The last rows below show Mr. M's responses, which reveal two chains: a typical or frequent scenario of drinking at home alone and a less frequent situation of dining at a restaurant with his son and getting into an argument.

The short-term, immediate consequences for drinking are often positive and therefore reinforce the behavior. In Mr. M's case, he felt happier immediately after the first drink, despite the fact that any euphoric effect of that first is, physiologically, likely to occur over a longer time frame. This would be illustrative of Mr. M's alcohol expectancies: He drinks with the expectation that he will feel better. According to the RP model, the probability of consuming more alcohol is thus increased.

Often, we have found that individuals in the early stage of RP treatment may have difficulties right away when asked to describe their antecedents—the thoughts (self-talk) or feelings that precede alcohol consumption. In such cases, asking about the consequences can be useful to fill in that unknown and we have found it helpful to ask the person a question such as "In general, on a day when you drink, what do you like about it?" If the person indicates they like getting intoxicated, we would re-ask the question: "Besides being intoxicated, what do you like about it?" The answer often helps the counselor and the individual clarify or identify the antecedents. Thus, when Mr. M reported feeling happier, it indicated he felt sad prior to taking the first drink on a typical day of drinking.

Antecedents →				Behavior →	Consequences	
Situations/thoughts +	Feelings +	Cues +	Urges →	First use on a typical day of substance use →	Immediate/Short-term (negative or positive)	Long-term (negative)
At home, alone, + thinking about my divorces	Depressed, bored	Remembers that there are beers in refrigerator	"A cold beer will help me forget my troubles"	First drink of beer	Feel happier, less sad (+)	Continues drinking six pack; feels ill, stomach upset (-)
Arguing with son at restaurant	Frustrated, feeling disrespected	Seeing others drinking	"I'll fix him. He hates it when I drink"	First cocktail	Calmed down (+) Son yells at him about drinking (-)	Has 3 more cocktails; embarrasses son (-) Falls down outside (-)

Figure 9.2. Substance use behavior chain.

Some short-term consequences can be negative as well. In Mr. M's case, his son yells at him when he sees him taking that first drink. All long-term consequences after that are always considered negative outcomes (e.g., feeling sick, falling down, fighting). The negative consequences recorded from the SAPE interview were used as reminders later in treatment after Mr. M was taught the coping skills to address his high-risk situations. In RP treatment, each client is provided with a wallet-sized consequences card and instructed to review it prior to taking a drink. When clients have learned appropriate coping skills for the antecedents to high-risk situations for drinking, but still feel the strong urge (self-statement) to drink, they are encouraged to review the consequences card and remember the steps for getting out of the situation.

For illustration purposes, we chose to describe how the RP model applied to Mr. M's use of alcohol. The pattern suggests two high-risk situations that lend themselves to training Mr. M in skills necessary to deal with each of the high-risk situations. For dealing with his feelings of loneliness, Mr. M would be taught cognitive behavioral approaches to recognize and modify negative thoughts before they progress further and the strong cue of the beer in the refrigerator becomes closer to the familiar action of drinking to forget his troubles. For the other situation involving the conflict with his son, if this is somewhat frequent (rather than a one-time occurrence), Mr. M. would be taught skills related to recognizing his triggers for anger and frustration and learning to be assertive rather than being either passive or the opposite (aggressive or confrontational).

Note that the focus on the antecedents and consequences is on the *first* drink on a typical day when consuming alcohol, not on subsequent, continued use. The goal is to use this information during the treatment modules to teach the client about his own frequent situations leading to drinking, then to teach the skills to cope with such situations as early in the chain as possible and well before the first drink is consumed.

We may also want to address Mr. M's misuse of medication. For misuse of legitimately prescribed medications, it is likely that many older adults are attempting to use the medication for the appropriate symptom but not following instructions for proper use. In Mr. M's case, overuse and doctor shopping were motivated by the need for relief from chronic pain, rather than by a desire to obtain medication for recreational purposes. Furthermore, we would need to take into consideration the pharmacokinetics and pharmacodynamics of prescription medications in older adults. Many medications take longer than alcohol for physiological effects to take place, and many medications have a longer half-life for complete metabolization or elimination from the system. Therefore, applying an RP model to Mr. M's medication misuse may require us to consider one of two strategies. The first strategy is to consider "taking a pill" as a parallel to consuming the first drink. If Mr. M takes a pain pill to escape feelings of anger, the focus would be similar to what is illustrated in Figure 9.2.

The second, alternative strategy of applying the RP model for medication misuse is to identify Mr. M's stated reason for consuming the medication on any given day. If he experiences pain flare-ups, we would inquire or have him log when these occur, the time of day, and the circumstances around that. This is similar to a published case example of an elderly woman abusing pain pills to alleviate frequent back pain flare-ups (Schonfeld, 1993). In this case, the B part of the chain was shifted to "pain flare-ups" that led her to consume more pain medications than prescribed. Additionally, the woman had arguments with the daughter, felt the pain flare-ups, and then took multiple pills in a short time.

Goal Setting

Once the information from the SAPE is completed, the final activity taught in Stage 1 is to identify a mutually acceptable goal with respect to substance use. In many treatment programs, success is defined as complete abstinence from the problem substance. However, if that were the only way to define success, there would be few successes, especially in outpatient treatment.

In the RP approach, using motivational interviewing approaches, the counselor negotiated with Mr. M on what he would like to accomplish with respect to alcohol use and separately regarding appropriate use of his prescribed medications. Using motivational interviewing, the therapist shaped this discussion to identify a goal that was both medically appropriate and acceptable to the client. The counselor educated Mr. M by discussing the definition of a standard drink and the recommended limits for a healthy older adult (i.e., no more than one drink per day). Given Mr. M's health problems and long history of problems with alcohol and pain medication, the counselor and Mr. M agreed on a goal of abstinence from alcohol, and a behavioral contract was written and signed by Mr. M and his lead clinician. In addition, he agreed to complete weekly alcohol self-monitoring logs and review those with the clinician.

For medication use, the goal was to use medications as prescribed, reduce dosages, and rely on a primary physician to ensure proper coordination of medications. To accomplish this, the clinician working with Mr. M developed a written behavioral contract and rehearsed questions that Mr. M could pose to his physician about the effectiveness of and his satisfaction with those medications.

Last, Mr. M and his primary counselor addressed family and social goals that if accomplished, would lead to improved quality of life. Mr. M's goals were to have improved relationships with family members, his most recent ex-wife, and with women in general.

Stage 2: Teaching the A-B-Cs

Once the components of Mr. M's behavior chain(s) were identified and goals were negotiated, the second stage of the RP model involved teaching him about his personal antecedents and consequences. The aim of this approach is to "take the mystery" out of his substance use so that he does not say, "I don't know why I drink so much." In this second stage, the counselor met with Mr. M to review the information transcribed from the SAPE interview, and then Mr. M entered into an A-B-Cs group (which can take either a group or an individual format).

In the A-B-Cs module, individuals are taught to recognize their own substance use chain first, by using simple examples provided in the exercises, then extended to their answers provided in responses to the SAPE questions. Quizzes and discussions provide tests for determining whether they have learned that information, an important step in ensuring that they will remember these as warning signs of potential future triggers for relapse.

Mr. M was taught how to complete a weekly log used to list events for each day and whether those events did or did not lead to an urge to drink or use other substances. An urge is not considered a biological event, but rather a "self-statement" such as "a cold beer will help me forget my troubles." Such a statement is the last component of the antecedents before taking that first drink and in effect would give Mr. M a rationale or permission to use the substance. He was instructed that if he experienced such an urge, he should record it on the log and indicate how he responded (i.e., did he consume alcohol, and if so, why? Or did he not use alcohol and why not?)

Despite Mr. M's long history of substance dependence, it should be noted that in diagramming the antecedents, the focus will not be on the long-term history, but instead the counselor will focus on recent and frequent events or behaviors that preceded recent substance use using a time frame of the 30 days preceding his last drink. Thus, for his drinking, the B (behavior) refers to the first drink or drug use, not prolonged or continued bouts of substance use thereafter. In the latter part of the chain, we focus on the C (consequences) for Mr. M to identify what happens after that first drink or use of a substance. Mr. M had to demonstrate his knowledge of his own short-term or immediate consequences that reinforced his taking the first drink. So, when he felt sad, he would report feeling happier immediately after that drink due to his expectancy of that positive effect. The negative consequences of the alcohol consumption, both short-term and long-term, listed on Mr. M's personalized consequences card were found to be useful prompts to avoid the unpleasant events or behaviors, or as clients have reported, a helpful reminder of what they stand to lose if they forget to use what they have learned in treatment.

Stage 3: Teaching the Skills to Prevent Relapse

The main part of the treatment in the RP model combines cognitive behavior therapy approaches that can be offered in formal outpatient and residential treatment programs (Benshoff, Koch, & Harrawood, 2003) with self-management approaches. Whether conducted in group or individual (one-on-one) treatment settings, these methods permit treatment plans to be tailored to each person's high-risk situations, in contrast to other treatment models (e.g., 12-step approaches) that are more likely to be the one-size-fits-all method that assumes everyone abuses substances in the same way and experiences similar problems.

Holder, Longabaugh, Miller, and Rubonis (1991) demonstrated that treatment programs focusing on social skills training, self-control training, and other behavioral interventions have higher rates of success and cost-effectiveness than other methods of treatment. Cognitive behavior therapy programs teach clients the skills necessary to recognize high-risk situations for substance use; interrupt or restructure the thoughts and situations that are likely to lead to substance use; and ultimately, prevent relapse. Fleming (2002) noted that the alcohol treatment field is moving away from a focus on abstinence and toward a harm-reduction public health paradigm.

Several publications by SAMHSA's CSAT promote these methods. The Treatment Improvement Protocol (TIP) #26 in *Substance Abuse Among Older Adults* (CSAT, 1998) provides expert panel consensus for identifying and treating substance abuse problems in older people. TIP #34 distinguishes between brief advice/intervention and brief therapies (CSAT, 1999) but is not specific to older people.

In this third stage of the treatment protocol, the counselor relied on self-management and cognitive behavioral approaches to teach Mr. M the skills necessary to address his individual high-risk situations in order to prevent relapse. Each module is a scripted lesson plan, containing lecture content, instructions for conducting behavior rehearsals, pretest and posttest quizzes and ratings of cognitive and behavioral rehearsals, and other exercises.

Table 9.1 presents the nine modules in the RP curriculum, beginning with the A-B-Cs module as a mandatory starting place. Each module contains a lesson plan, goals for the session, required visual aid, a complete script for the session, and exercises and quizzes to test the client's retention of the information learned. As shown in the table, a variety of skills are taught such as thought-stopping, covert assertion, cognitive restructuring, and problem-solving skills through didactic and experiential exercises, including behavior rehearsals. In rehearsals, clients practice skills in a nonthreatening, simulated situation that resembles a real situation likely to occur outside of the treatment setting, and that has led to drinking or drug use in the past (i.e., the

TABLE 9.1
Description of the CBT/Self-Management Modules

Module	Content	Methods used
A-B-Cs of substance use	• Identify personal high-risk situations • Identify antecedents and consequences for high-risk situations • Diagram personal drinking behavior chain	• Functional analysis of behavior using general examples • Self-monitor urges by completing a weekly log
Social pressure	• How to refuse an offer of a drink • How to say no to a persistent "pusher" without being aggressive	• Behavior rehearsal/role plays • Basic assertiveness and communication skills
At home and alone	• How to avoid being lonely and becoming sad • Identify pleasant events and alternative behaviors	• Thought-stopping • Cognitive restructuring • Covert behavior rehearsal
Thoughts and negative emotions	• Identify negative thoughts and feelings preceding drinking • Identify positive self-statements	• Thought-stopping • Cognitive restructuring • Covert assertion
Anxiety and tension	• Identify signs of tension building • Interrupt negative, ruminative thoughts • Begin to relax • Generate alternative solutions and try them out	• Brief relaxation • Thought-stopping • Cognitive restructuring • Covert assertion • Problem Solving Skills
Anger and frustration	• Appropriate assertiveness skills rather than aggressive or passive behaviors • DESC Model (Describe objectionable behavior to the other person, Express feelings, Specify changes, and indicate beneficial Consequences)	• Thought-stopping • Cognitive restructuring • Covert assertion
Controlling substance use cues	• CARD model: Identify behaviors that Compete with drinking, Avoid cues, Rearrange your life, Dispose of cues)	• Covert behavior rehearsal
Coping with urges	• Urges are considered self-statements that give one permission to drink • CRASH Model—(remember Consequences, Remove from situation, find incompatible Activity, use Skills learned, call for Help)	• Covert behavior rehearsal
Preventing a slip from becoming a relapse	• Make a positive statement about stopping • Get out of the situation or get rid of the alcohol • Call for help	• Covert behavior rehearsal

high-risk situation). In treatment, Mr. M learned about situations that triggered his anger, such as having his son yell at him if he thought Mr. M had drank alcohol. He learned ways to be assertive, without being either passive or aggressive, then with behavior rehearsals, practiced those in the groups. Similarly, for addressing negative moods such as depression and loneliness, Mr. M rehearsed aloud in groups steps he would take to interrupt ruminating thoughts and emphasize more positive and accurate statements (i.e., a covert assertion method in which thoughts are replaced).

Given the previous research on older adults in treatment, much of the RP curriculum emphasizes skills for addressing negative emotional states. Such skills include recognizing inaccurate, ruminative thoughts and using thought-stopping to interrupt ruminations, followed by covert assertion (i.e., replacing those thoughts with positive and more accurate self-statements). Other modules focus on social pressure, managing feelings of anger and frustration over interactions with other people. General problem-solving skills are also taught in several of the modules.

Self-management techniques with the RP model are designed to teach behavioral principles for managing substance use behavior (Kanfer, 1975). First, self-monitoring is taught by having each client complete logs that are later reviewed by the counselor, who in turn provides feedback aimed at preventing future slips or relapses. Second, clients have homework assignments such as contacting a drinking or drug-use hotline to find out what the counselors would do if the individual experiences a slip. Third, a therapist might use *behavior contracting*, an agreement that spells out the expected behavioral goal and the consequences should the behavior occur or not occur. Clients also learn to use self-reinforcement, such as rewarding oneself for engaging in a preferred nondrinking activity.

It is important to rehearse with clients what to do if they experience a slip. Staff members should encourage clients so that they feel comfortable enough to report a slip or a relapse without fear of being labeled or accused of failure. A lapse actually becomes a learning experience as counselor and client review the event and diagram the components of the behavior chain preceding the slip. Once diagrammed, the skills are rehearsed.

Determining Readiness for Discharge

Discharge from treatment should be based on each client's ability to demonstrate that he has actually learned the skills and knowledge taught within treatment, as well as the ability to maintain his treatment goal (limit of no more than one drink per day or complete abstinence). In the RP curriculum there are quizzes, exercises, and rehearsals that are rated so that the client can demonstrate what was learned and what to do if a high-risk situation is encountered. Clients who have difficulties attaining a goal, such as complete abstinence, should negotiate with their counselors to identify a less difficult goal, such as no more than one drink on any occasion. Second, each individual participating in the RP treatment must receive passing scores or ratings on quizzes or behavior rehearsals. If the client cannot demonstrate acceptable performance on these two criteria, remediation or one-on-one tutoring may be required until she or he does so.

Third, each client must demonstrate the ability to diagram his or her personal drinking behavior chain and high-risk situations. When the client can do so, and can demonstrate competence in the skills learned, discharge planning can begin.

Mr. M's Outcomes

Mr. M successfully completed the A-B-Cs module and the self-management skills training. Key to his high-risk situations were identification of feelings of loneliness and depression and learning how to become engaged in social activities he would enjoy that also did not involve drinking. He learned how to deal with his feelings of anger and frustration, often focused on how to better communicate with his son, so that such situations did not lead to drinking episodes. Quiz and homework assignments indicated that he attained the knowledge about his personal substance use behavior chains as outlined in Figure 9.2. He also participated in a men's group, in a group titled "Enjoying the Golden Years," and in an individual therapy session during his stay at Senior Hope Counseling.

Mr. M reported to staff how comfortable he felt attending groups in which other clients were similar in age and life experience. He felt valued, respected, and able to sit in a group with none of the foul language often experienced when participating in mixed-age treatment, so that he was comfortable sharing his struggles with alcohol and medications. Mr. M continued to complete weekly logs to record any urges to consume alcohol and whether or not urges were followed by a drink.

With respect to management of prescription medications, Mr. M learned how concomitant use of alcohol and medications could adversely affect his emotional and physical well-being. He began discussions with his physician about his concurrent use of alcohol and informed the physician about the severity of his shoulder and back pain as well as past attempts to doctor shop. Mr. M enrolled in a pain management clinic, and the primary clinician and the prescribing physician both contacted the clinic to increase communication and provide support to help Mr. M adhere to an appropriate medication regimen to control his chronic pain. As a result, Mr. M learned how painkillers were actually causing many of the symptoms he experienced, including muscle spasm, muscle twitching, muscle pain, diarrhea, constipation, sleep disturbance, and a general inability to communicate adequately with the important people around him. He also found alternative ways of thinking and behaving in order to adhere to the regimen, to not rush to take extra painkillers, and to not seek other physicians.

Following discharge from treatment, Mr. M began attending AA and NA. He reported that he remained abstinent and rarely noted the urge to drink on the weekly logs. At discharge, Mr. M was able to discontinue all opioid medications and manage his pain through the nonaddictive medications prescribed by his physician. The pain clinic staff helped by teaching him how to use a transcutaneous electrical nerve stimulation unit. He also received acupuncture treatments. Mr. M reported that because he took these steps, he no longer sought to overmedicate or shop for doctors who would add to his prescriptions.

In the goal-setting stage early in treatment, Mr. M expressed a desire to improve relationships with family, his ex-wife, his adult children, and with women with whom he could socialize. He reported that he accomplished these goals using the skills he learned at Senior Hope Counseling. The positive feedback and support from his family and the people around him further encouraged him to maintain his aftercare plan and continue logging his urges to drink. He also found himself spending time with women who did not use alcohol or drugs. He reported improved relations with his last ex-wife and his children from his last marriage and was dating a woman who he felt was "healthy." Mr. M attributed these positive outcomes to the skills he learned in the program. At discharge he reported that, thanks to these acquired skills, he became attracted to "healthier" women and experienced improved relations with his children.

CONCLUSION

In this chapter, we described age-specific issues that affect the treatment of older adults. These include challenges in identifying problems and meeting diagnostic criteria. We then explained how the RP model, an evidence-based treatment modality, was applied to older adults to address their substance misuse.

A number of aging-related issues differentiate older adults' problems from those of their younger counterparts. First, in contrast to younger adults, who often abuse substances in response to interpersonal antecedents (e.g., social pressure, partying, conflicts with other people), research has shown that older adults with substance abuse problems experience a higher incidence of antecedents that are intrapersonal in nature (Schonfeld et al., 1995). These include negative emotional states, feelings of loneliness or boredom, pain from illness or injury, loss of social support, and so on. Second, when considering group treatment, older adults often report a greater level of comfort and perhaps treatment compliance when entered into elder-specific treatment rather than being in mixed-age treatment. Third, treatment planning focusing on identifying high-risk situations for substance use and tailoring treatment to address those situations is likely to reduce lapses or relapses. Fourth, prescribing physicians and substance abuse treatment staff need to collaborate to prevent relapse in medication misuse among older adults. Such misuse is often an attempt by the older adult to manage the symptoms (e.g., pain) for which the medications are legitimately prescribed. This is very different from the majority of young adults, who obtain medications illegally through "pill mills" and doctor shopping in order to resell them for profit or use them for recreational purposes.

The RP curriculum we described can be adapted for any age group or for various substance use problems. The benefit of the approach is that it aims not only for changes in substance use but also for changes in the behaviors that are likely to trigger misuse.

REFERENCES

Alzheimer's Association. (2014). *Korsakoff syndrome*. Retrieved from http://www.alz.org/dementia/downloads/topicsheet_korsakoff.pdf

American Geriatrics Society 2012 Beers Criteria Update Expert Panel. (2012). American Geriatrics Society Updated Beers Criteria for Potentially Inappropriate Medication Use in Older Adults. *Journal of the American Geriatrics Society, 60*, 616–631. doi:10.1111/j.1532-5415.2012.03923.x

American Psychiatric Association. (2000). *Diagnostic and statistical manual of mental disorders* (4th ed., text rev.). Washington, DC: Author.

American Psychiatric Association. (2013). *Diagnostic and statistical manual of mental disorders* (5th ed.). Washington, DC: Author.

Benshoff, J. J., Koch, D. S., & Harrawood, L. K. (2003). Substance abuse and the elderly: Unique issues and concerns. *Journal of Rehabilitation, 69*(2), 43–48.

Blazer, D. G., & Wu, L. T. (2009). The epidemiology of at-risk and binge drinking among middle-aged and elderly community adults: National Survey on Drug Use and Health. *The American Journal of Psychiatry, 166*, 1162–1169. doi:10.1176/appi.ajp.2009.09010016

Carstensen, L. L., Rychtarik, R. G., & Prue, D. M. (1985). Behavioral treatment of the geriatric alcohol abuser: A long term follow-up study. *Addictive Behaviors, 10*, 307–311. doi:10.1016/0306-4603(85)90012-7

Center for Substance Abuse Treatment, Substance Abuse and Mental Health Services Administration, U.S. Department of Health and Human Services. (1998).

Substance abuse among older adults (HHS Publication No. [SMA] 12-3918). Rockville, MD: Author. Retrieved from http://www.ncbi.nlm.nih.gov/books/NBK64422

Center for Substance Abuse Treatment, Substance Abuse and Mental Health Services Administration, U.S. Department of Health and Human Services. (1999). *Brief Interventions and Brief Therapies for Substance Abuse: Treatment Improvement Protocol (TIP) Series 34* (DHHS Publication No. [SMA] 99-3353). Rockville, MD: Author. Retrieved from http://store.samhsa.gov/product/TIP-34-Brief-Interventions-and-Brief-Therapies-for-Substance-Abuse/SMA12-3452

Center for Substance Abuse Treatment, Substance Abuse and Mental Health Services Administration, U.S. Department of Health and Human Services. (2005). *Substance abuse relapse prevention for older adults: A group treatment approach* (DHHS Publication No. [SMA] 05-4053). Rockville MD: Author. Retrieved from http://store.samhsa.gov/product/Substance-Abuse-Relapse-Prevention-for-Older-Adults-A-Group-Treatment-Approach/SMA05-4053

Colliver, J. D., Compton, W. M., Gfroerer, T. C., & Condon, T. (2006). Projecting drug use among baby-boomers in 2020. *Annals of Epidemiology, 16,* 257–265. doi:10.1016/j.annepidem.2005.08.003

Compton, W. M., Dawson, D. A., Goldstein, R. B., & Grant, B. F. (2013). Crosswalk between DSM–IV dependence and DSM–5 substance use disorders for opioids, cannabis, cocaine and alcohol. *Drug and Alcohol Dependence, 132,* 387–390. doi:10.1016/j.drugalcdep.2013.02.036

Dupree, L. W., Broskowski, H., & Schonfeld, L. (1984). The Gerontology Alcohol Project: A behavioral treatment program for elderly alcohol abusers. *The Gerontologist, 24,* 510–516. doi:10.1093/geront/24.5.510

Fleming, M. (2002). Identification and treatment of alcohol use disorders in the elderly. In A. M. Gurnack, R. Atkinson, & N. J. Osgood (Eds.), *Treating alcohol and drug abuse in the elderly* (pp. 85–108). New York, NY: Springer.

Graham, K., Brett, P. J., & Baron, J. (1997). A harm reduction approach to treating older adults: The clients speak. In D. M. R. P. G. Erickson, Y. W. Cheung, & P. A. O'Hare (Eds.), *Harm reduction: A new direction for drug policies and programs* (pp. 428–452). Toronto, Ontario, Canada: University of Toronto Press.

Gupta, S., & Warner, J. (2008). Alcohol-related dementia: A 21st-century silent epidemic? *The British Journal of Psychiatry, 193,* 351–353. doi:10.1192/bjp.bp.108.051425

Holder, H., Longabaugh, R., Miller, W. R., & Rubonis, A. V. (1991). The cost effectiveness of treatment for alcoholism: A first approximation. *Journal of Studies on Alcohol, 52,* 517–540.

Kanfer, F. (1975). Self-management methods. In F. H. Kanfer & A. P. Goldstein (Eds.), *Helping people change: A textbook of methods* (pp. 309–355). New York, NY: Pergamon Press, Inc.

Kofoed, L. L., Tolson, R., Atkinson, R. M., Toth, R., & Turner, J. (1987). Treatment compliance of older alcoholics: An elder-specific approach is superior to "mainstreaming." *Journal of Studies on Alcohol, 48,* 47–51.

Marlatt, G. A. (1976). The Drinking Profile: A questionnaire for the behavioral assessment of alcoholism. In E. J. Mash & L. G. Terdal (Eds.), *Behavior therapy assessment: Diagnosis, design, and evaluation* (pp. 121–137). New York, NY: Springer.

Sabia, S., Elbaz, A., Britton, A., Bell, A., Dugravot, M., Shipley, M., Kivimaki, M., & Singh-Manoux, A. (2014). Alcohol consumption and cognitive decline in early old age. *Neurology, 82*, 332–339. doi:10.1212/WNL.0000000000000063

Schonfeld, L. (1993). Covert assertion as a method for coping with pain and pain related behaviors. *Clinical Gerontologist, 12*(1), 17–29. doi:10.1300/J018v12n01_03

Schonfeld, L., Dupree, L. W., Dickson-Fuhrmann, E., Royer, C. M., McDermott, C. H., Rosansky, J. S., . . . Jarvik, L. F. (2000). Cognitive-behavioral treatment of older veterans with substance abuse problems. *Journal of Geriatric Psychiatry and Neurology, 13*, 124–129. doi:10.1177/089198870001300305

Schonfeld, L., Dupree, L. W., & Rohrer, G. E. (1995). Age-specific differences between younger and older alcohol abusers. *Journal of Clinical Geropsychology, 1*(3), 219–227.

Schonfeld, L., King-Kallimanis, B. L., Duchene, D. M., Etheridge, R. L., Herrera, J. R., Barry, K. L., & Lynn, N. (2010). Screening and brief intervention for substance misuse among older adults: The Florida BRITE Project. *American Journal of Public Health, 100*(1), 108–114. doi:10.2105/AJPH.2008.149534

Substance Abuse and Mental Health Services Administration, U.S. Department of Health & Human Services. (2006). *DASIS Report. Issue 17. Older Adult Admissions: 2003*. Rockville, MD: Author. Retrieved from http://www.samhsa.gov/data/2k6/olderAdultsTX/olderAdultsTX.htm

Substance Abuse and Mental Health Services Administration, U.S. Department of Health & Human Services. (2010). *The NSDUH report: Substance use among American Indian or Alaska Native adults*. Rockville, MD: Author. Retrieved from http://www.samhsa.gov/data/2k10/182/AmericanIndian.htm

Substance Abuse and Mental Health Services Administration, U.S. Department of Health & Human Services. (2011). *Results from the 2010 National Survey on Drug Use and Health: Summary of National Findings*. (HHS Publication No. SMA 11-4658). Rockville, MD: Author. Retrieved from http://oas.samhsa.gov/NSDUH/2k10NSDUH/2k10Results.htm

Substance Abuse and Mental Health Services Administration, U.S. Department of Health & Human Services. (2012). *Treatment Episode Data Set (TEDS): 2000–2010. National Admissions to Substance Abuse Treatment Services*. Rockville, MD: Author. Retrieved from http://www.samhsa.gov/data/2k12/TEDS2010N/TEDS2010NChp3.htm

Substance Abuse and Mental Health Services Administration, U.S. Department of Health & Human Services. (2014). *Relapse prevention therapy*. Retrieved from http://www.nrepp.samhsa.gov/ViewIntervention.aspx?id=97

U.S. Office of Disability. (2014). *Substance abuse and disability*. Retrieved from http://www.hhs.gov/od/about/fact_sheets/substanceabuse.html

ADDITIONAL RESOURCES
FOR CLINICIANS

In this section, we provide a list of resources for readers who are interested in learning more about the interventions and information provided in this book. It is a compilation of resources each author recommends, but it does not constitute a comprehensive list of all resources in the field.

COGNITIVE BEHAVIOR THERAPY (CBT)
AND BEHAVIORAL ACTIVATION

Client Self-Help Books

Addis, M., & Martell, C. (2004). *Overcoming depression one step at a time*. Oakland, CA: New Harbinger.

Burns, D. (1999). *The feeling good handbook* (Rev. ed.). New York, NY: Penguin.

Craske, G. M., & Barlow, D. H. (2006). *Mastery of your anxiety and worry* (2nd ed.). New York, NY: Oxford University Press.

Gilbert, P. (2009). *Overcoming depression: A self-help guide using cognitive behavioral techniques* (3rd ed.). New York, NY: Basic Books.

Greenberger, D., & Padesky, C. (1995). *Mind over mood: A cognitive therapy treatment manual for clients*. New York, NY: Guilford Press.

Lewinsohn, P., Munoz, R., Youngren, M., & Zeiss, A. (1992). *Control your depression*. New York, NY: Simon & Schuster.

Wright, J., Basco, M., & Thase, M. (2006). *Learning cognitive–behavior therapy: An illustrated guide*. Washington, DC: American Psychiatric Association.

Books for Clinicians

Craske, G. M. (2010). *Cognitive–behavioral therapy*. Washington, DC: American Psychological Association.

Gallagher-Thompson, D., Steffen, A. M., & Thompson, L. W. (2008). *Handbook of behavioral and cognitive therapies with older adults*. New York, NY: Springer. doi:10.1007/978-0-387-72007-4

Laidlaw, K., Thompson, L. W., Dick-Siskin, L., & Gallagher-Thompson, D. (2003). *Cognitive behaviour therapy with older people*. New York, NY: Wiley. doi:10.1002/9780470713402

Scogin, F., & Shah, A. (2012). *Making evidence-based psychological treatments work with older adults*. Washington, DC: American Psychological Association. doi:10.1037/13753-000

Sorocco, K. H., & Lauderdale, S. (2011). *Cognitive behavior therapy with older adults: Innovations across care settings*. New York, NY: Springer.

Sorocco, K. H., & Lauderdale, S. (2011). *Implementing CBT for older adults*. New York, NY: Springer.

Stanley, M. A., Diefenbach, G. J., & Hopko, D. R. (2004). Cognitive behavioral treatment for older adults with generalized anxiety disorder: A therapist manual for primary care settings. *Behavior Modification, 28*, 73–117. doi:10.1097/JGP.0b013e3182546167

Free Videos

Center for Cognitive and Behavioral Therapy of Greater Columbus. [ccbtcolumbus]. (2010, June 23). *Behavioral activation for depression* [with K. Arnold]. Retrieved from http://www.youtube.com/watch?v=Dp6i3GUasqQ

Cognitive Behavior Associates. [CognitiveBT]. (2008, September 9). *CBT for depression* [with J. Becker]. Retrieved from http://www.youtube.com/watch?v=Usnlzh8Bneg

Padesky, C. [Christine A. Padesky, PhD]. (2011, January 31). *Padesky on CBT case conceptualization*. Retrieved from http://www.youtube.com/watch?v=K0mfVEVUAV0

Psychotherapy.net. [PsychotherapyNet]. (2009, April 1). Meichenbaum cognitive–behavioral therapy video [with R. Meichenbaum]. Retrieved from http://www.youtube.com/watch?v=8cK4xdZvHUM

Psychotherapy Videos and DVDs. [PsychotherapyDVDs]. (2009, October 11). *CBT: Work on the continuum*. Retrieved from http://www.youtube.com/watch?v=odB7j_zH5Rs

DVDs for Purchase

American Psychological Association. (Producer). (2005). *Systems of psychotherapy video series: Cognitive therapy* [with J. Beck] [DVD]. Available from http://www.apa.org/pubs/videos/4310736.aspx

American Psychological Association. (Producer). (2006). *Cognitive–behavior therapy for depression video series: Activity scheduling* [with J. B. Persons, J. Davidson, & M. A. Tompkins] [DVD]. Available from http://www.apa.org/pubs/videos/4310748.aspx

American Psychological Association. (Producer). (2007). *Cognitive–behavior therapy for depression video series: Structure of the therapy session* [with J. Davidson, J. B. Persons, & M. A. Tompkins] [DVD]. Available from http://www.apa.org/pubs/videos/4310790.aspx

American Psychological Association. (Producer). (2007). *Cognitive–behavior therapy for depression video series: Using the thought record* [with J. Davidson, J. B. Persons, & M. A. Tompkins] [DVD]. Available from http://www.apa.org/pubs/videos/4310789.aspx

Padesky, C. (Producer). (n.d.) *Cognitive therapy training on discs series* [DVD]. Available from http://store.padesky.com/

Treatment Manuals

Addis, M., & Martell, C. (2004). *Overcoming depression one step at a time*. Oakland, CA: New Harbinger.

Beck, A., Rush, A., Shaw, B., & Emery, G. (1979). *Cognitive therapy of depression*. New York, NY: Guilford Press.

Beck, J. S. (2011). *Cognitive behavior therapy: Basics and beyond* (2nd ed.). New York, NY: Guilford Press.

Gilson, M., Freeman, A., Yates, M., & Freeman, S. (2009). *Overcoming depression: A cognitive therapy approach workbook (treatments that work)*. New York, NY: Oxford University Press.

Martell, C., Addis, M., & Jacobson, N. (2001). *Depression in context: Strategies for guided action*. New York, NY: Norton.

Martell, C., Dimidjian, S., & Herman-Dunn, R. (2010). *Behavioral activation for depression: A clinician's guide*. New York, NY: Guilford Press.

CBT Organizations and Training Workshops

Academy of Cognitive Therapy (http://www.academyofct.org): Certification in Cognitive Therapy

The American Institute for Cognitive Therapy (http://www.cognitivetherapynyc.com): Weekend Workshops

Association for Behavioral and Cognitive Therapies (http://www.abct.org)

Atlanta Center for Cognitive Therapy (http://www.cognitiveatlanta.com): Professional training

Beck Institute for Cognitive Behavior Therapy (http://www.beckinstitute.org): CBT Training and Workshops

Massachusetts General Hospital's Psychiatry Academy: The Fundamentals of CBT, An Interactive Online Course (http://www.mghcme.org/cbt)

University of Pennsylvania—Center for Cognitive Therapy (http://www.med.upenn.edu/cct/index.html): Cognitive Therapy Training Program

Stanford School of Medicine, Stanford Geriatric Education Center (http://sgec.stanford.edu/training/behavior-activation.html): Training materials for using behavioral activation to reduce depression in older adults

Other Resources

Evidence-based behavioral practice website: http://www.ebbp.org/skillsBasedResources.html

INTERPERSONAL PSYCHOTHERAPY

Books for Clinicians

Frank, K., & Levenson, J. C. (2010). *Interpersonal psychotherapy*. Washington, DC: American Psychological Association.

Miller, M. (2009). *A clinician's guide to interpersonal therapy for late life*. New York, NY: Oxford University Press.

DVDs for Purchase

American Psychological Association. (Producer). (2007). *Clinical geropsychology video series: Interpersonal therapy for older adults with depression* [with G. A. Hinrichsen] [DVD]. Available from http://www.apa.org/pubs/videos/4310796.aspx

Treatment Manuals

Miller, M. (2009). *Clinician's guide to interpersonal psychotherapy in late life: Helping cognitively impaired or depressed elders and their caregivers*. New York, NY: Oxford University Press.

Organizations and Training Workshops

The Interpersonal Therapy Institute: https://iptinstitute.com/ipt-certification-process/

PROBLEM-SOLVING TREATMENT (PST)

Client Self-Help Books

National Network of PST Clinicians, Trainers, & Researchers. *Materials*. Retrieved from http://pstnetwork.ucsf.edu/materials

Books for Clinicians

D'Zurilla, T., & Nezu, A. M. (2006). *Problem-solving therapy: A positive approach to clinical intervention* (3rd ed.). New York, NY: Springer.

Nezu, A. M., Nezu, C. M., & D'Zurilla (2012). *Problem-solving therapy: A treatment manual*. New York, NY: Springer.

Free Videos

UCSFPSTTTraining. (2012, October 17). *PST intro training session*. Retrieved from http://youtu.be/wpSIwt6G-Tw

UCSFPSTTTraining. (2013, June 27). *PST mid session Part 1*. Retrieved from http://youtu.be/5jOllifW8sE

UCSFPSTTTraining. (2012, October 17). *PST mid session Part 2*. Retrieved from http://youtu.be/ishiAyXXXPU

UCSFPSTTTraining. (2013, May 30). *PST termination session Part 1*. Retrieved from http://youtu.be/DgH_XO7b9-4

UCSFPSTTTraining. (2013, May 30). *PST termination session Part 2*. Retrieved from http://youtu.be/-AhwhCfM_Ss

Treatment Manuals

Areán, P. A., Raue, P., & Julian, L. (2011). *Social problem-solving therapy for depression and executive dysfunction*. San Francisco, CA: The Over-60 Research Group, University of California. Retrieved from http://pstnetwork.ucsf.edu/sites/pstnetwork.ucsf.edu/files/documents/Social%20Problem%20Solving%20Therapy%20ED.Final_.pdf

Hegel, M. T., & Areán, P. A. (2011). *Problem-solving treatment for primary care (PST–PC): A treatment manual for depression*. San Francisco, CA: The Over-60 Research Group, University of California. Retrieved from http://pstnetwork.ucsf.edu/sites/pstnetwork.ucsf.edu/files/documents/Pst-PC%20Manual.pdf

Hegel, M. T., & Areán, P. A. (2011). *PST–PC appendix*. San Francisco, CA: The Over-60 Research Group, University of California. Retrieved from http://pstnetwork.ucsf.edu/sites/pstnetwork.ucsf.edu/files/documents/PST-PC%20APPENDIX.pdf

The Over-60 Research Group, University of California, San Francisco. (2007). *Problem-solving therapy for late-life depression*. San Francisco, CA: Author. Retrieved from http://pstnetwork.ucsf.edu/sites/pstnetwork.ucsf.edu/files/documents/PST%20manual%20NEW%202012.pdf

Organizations and Certification Programs for Clinicians

National Network of PST Clinician, Trainers and Researchers: http://pstnetwork.ucsf.edu

University of Washington AIMS Center: http://aims.uw.edu/

RELAXATION THERAPY

Client Self-Help Books

Davis, M., McKay, M., & Eshelman, E. R. (2008). *The relaxation & stress reduction workbook* (6th ed.). Oakland, CA: New Harbinger.

MOTIVATIONAL INTERVIEWING

Books for Clinicians

Hettema, J., Steele, J., & Miller, W. R. (2005). Motivational interviewing. *Annual Review of Clinical Psychology, 1*, 91–111. doi:10.1146/annurev.clinpsy.1.102803.143833

Miller, W. R., & Rollnick, S. (2012). *Motivational interviewing: Helping people change* (3rd ed.). New York, NY: Guilford Press.

National Institute on Drug Abuse. (2012). *Principles of drug addiction and treatment: A research-based guide* (3rd ed.). Bethesda, MD: National Institutes of Health.

Rollnick, S., Miller, W. R., & Butler, C. C. (2007). *Motivational interviewing in health-care*. New York, NY: Guilford Press.

Free Videos

Institute for Research, Education, and Training in Addictions. [TheIRETA channel]. (2013, June 18). *Motivational interviewing—A good example—Alan Lyme*. Retrieved from https://www.youtube.com/watch?v=67I6g1I7Zao

Oregon Geriatric Education Center. (2013, December 31). *Using motivational interviewing-based skills and strategies with older adults at risk for falls*. Retrieved from https://www.youtube.com/watch?v=IZR4Njufxs4

Treatment Manuals

Online Motivational Interviewing Training and Clinical Resources

Center for Evidence-Based Practices, Case Western Reserve University: http://www.centerforebp.case.edu/practices/mi

Center for Integrated Health Solutions: http://www.integration.samhsa.gov/clinical-practice/motivational-interviewing

Motivational Interviewing: http://www.motivationalinterview.org/

SAMHSA–HRSA

Substance Abuse and Mental Health Services Administration (SAMHSA) Co-Occurring Disorders: http://www.samhsa.gov/co-occurring/topics/training/change.aspx

Training Resources

Motivational Interviewing Network of Trainers (MINT): http://www.motivationalinterviewing.org/

Motivational Interviewing: http://www.motivationalinterview.org

Resources for Clinicians, Agency Administrators, Trainers, and Program Evaluators

Substance Abuse and Mental Health Services Administration. (1999). *SAMHSA Treatment Improvement Protocol (TIP) 35: Enhancing motivation for change in substance abuse treatment* (DHHS Publication No. 99–3354). Rockville, MD: U.S. Department of Health and Human Services. Retrieved from http://lib.adai.washington.edu/clearinghouse/downloads/TIP-35-Enhancing-Motivation-for-Change-in-Substance-Abuse-Treatment-59.pdf

SCREENING, BRIEF INTERVENTION, AND REFERRAL TO TREATMENT (SBIRT)

Free Videos

SBIRT Institute. (2011, March 2.) *SBIRT for alcohol use: Older man*. Retrieved from https://www.youtube.com/watch?v=XIi_ImmFafQ

Treatment Manuals

SAMHSA Clinical Practice Tool: http://www.integration.samhsa.gov/clinical-practice/sbirt

Organizations and Workshops

SAMHSA: Screening, Brief Intervention, and Referral to Treatment: http://www.samhsa.gov/prevention/SBIRT/index.aspx

HealtheKnowledge.org: http://www.healtheknowledge.org/

Clinical Tools, Inc.'s, SBIRT Training: Clinical Skills Training for Substance Use Problems: http://www.sbirttraining.com/

SBIRT online development courses, Center for Applied Behavioral Health Policy, Arizona State University: http://cabhp.asu.edu/professional-development/sbirt-development/sbirt-online

Other SBIRT Resources

UCLA Integrated Substance Abuse Programs and the Pacific Southwest Addiction Technology Transfer Center's *The World of SBIRT* website: http://worldofsbirt.wordpress.com/

TREATMENT LOCATORS

SAMHSA Behavioral Health Treatment Services Locator: http://findtreatment.samhsa.gov/
SAMHSA Treatment Referral Helpline:
   1-800-662-HELP (4357)
   1-800-487-4889 (TDD)
Anxiety Disorders Association of America: http://www.adaa.org

RESEARCH AND TRAINING SITES

Late-Life Anxiety Research Program, Baylor College of Medicine, Department of Psychiatry and Behavioral Sciences: http://www.bcm.edu/departments/psychiatry-and-behavioral-sciences

INDEX

and screening, brief intervention, and referral to treatment for substance abuse, 203

Cognitive training games, 8

Comas-Díaz, L., 61

Communication analysis, 76–77

Comorbidities
    with generalized anxiety disorder, 105, 121
    with substance use disorders, 197

Competencies, 13. *See also* Cultural competence; Pikes Peak model for geropsychology

Compton, W. M., 213

Content affect, 76–77

Contextual adult life span theory for adapting psychotherapy (CALTAP), 54, 61

Cook, J. M., 152

Coon, D. W., 51

CoPGTP (Council of Professional Geropsychology Training Programs), 23–24

COPPES (California Older Person's Pleasant Events Schedule), 57

Cornelius, T. L., 139

Coronary heart disease, 104

Council for Professional Training in Geropsychology, 16, 23

Council of Professional Geropsychology Training Programs (CoPGTP), 23–24

Cuijpers, P., 6

Cultural competence, 62, 147–148

Cultural considerations
    behavioral activation therapy for depression, 60–62
    cognitive behavior therapy for depression, 60–62
    EBT for generalized anxiety disorder, 119
    exposure therapy for late-life trauma, 146–149
    interpersonal psychotherapy for depression, 79
    motivational interviewing for alcohol and drug misuse, 174–175
    problem-solving therapy for depression, 96–97
    relapse prevention for substance use disorders, 215–216

screening, brief intervention, and referral to treatment for substance abuse, 202–203

Current Opioid Misuse Measure, 194

Dai, Y., 61

Danckwerts, A., 151

DAST (Drug Abuse Screening Test), 192–193

Dawson, D. A., 213

Dementia, 105, 150, 217

Depression, late-life
    behavioral activation therapy for. *See* Behavioral activation therapy for late-life depression
    cognitive behavior therapy for. *See* Cognitive behavior therapy for late-life depression
    comorbidity with anxiety disorders, 105, 121
    interpersonal psychotherapy for. *See* Interpersonal psychotherapy for late-life depression
    problem-solving therapy for. *See* Problem-solving therapy for late-life depression

Diagnostic and Statistical Manual of Mental Disorders (*DSM–5*)
    current changes to, 7
    generalized anxiety disorder criteria in, 119
    PTSD criteria in, 133–135
    substance use disorder criteria in, 168, 195, 212–213

Diagnostic and Statistical Manual of Mental Disorders (*DSM–IV–TR*)
    PTSD criteria in, 134
    substance use disorder criteria in, 195, 212–213

Dickinson, K. C., 202

Dick-Siskin, L., 51

Diefenbach, G. J., 104

Dimidjian, S., 56

Disabilities, patients with
    and behavioral activation therapy, 62–63
    and cognitive behavior therapy, 62–63
    and exposure therapy for late-life trauma, 149–150
    and interpersonal psychotherapy, 79

ABOUT THE EDITOR

Patricia A. Areán, PhD, is a professor in the department of psychiatry at the University of California, San Francisco, and a licensed clinical psychologist. Dr. Areán is an international expert on the effectiveness of behavioral interventions for mood disorders, in particular on adapting these interventions for a variety of health and mental health settings (primary care medicine, assisted living, social service, mental health) and more recently on mobile health applications. Since 1994, she has published more than 100 peer-reviewed articles on these topics and has been funded by the Substance Abuse and Mental Health Services Administration, National Institute of Mental Health (NIMH), National Institute on Aging, National Institute of Diabetes and Digestive and Kidney Diseases, and the Hartford Foundation. She is currently funded by NIMH to study the effectiveness of brain games and mobile health apps on mood. Dr. Areán's work has won national recognition, resulting in an early career award from the American Psychological Association, a mid-career Award from the National Institutes of Health for her work on disseminating evidence-based practices, and the Award for Achievements in Diversity in Mental Health from the American Association of Geriatric Psychiatry. Dr. Areán currently leads an interdisciplinary research team of researchers from diverse backgrounds, including social work, nursing, psychiatry, family and general medicine, medical sociology, and clinical psychology.